ECG
Board Review and
Study Guide

Part 2
Sample ECGs and Answers

By
James H. O'Keefe, Jr., MD, FACC
Associate Professor of Medicine
University of Missouri, Kansas City Medical School
Clinical Nuclear Cardiologist
Mid America Heart Institute
Kansas City, Missouri

Stephen C. Hammill, MD, FACC
Professor of Medicine
Director, Electrocardiography and
Electrophysiology Laboratories
Mayo Clinic
Rochester, Minnesota

Mark R. Zolnick, MD, FACC
Clinical Instructor of Medicine
Jefferson Medical College
Philadelphia, Pennsylvania;
Medical Director of Coronary Intensive Care Unit
Medical Center of Delaware
Newark, Delaware

David M. Steinhaus, MD, FACC
Associate Professor of Medicine
University of Missouri, Kansas City Medical School
Co-Director, Electrophysiology Laboratory
Mid America Heart Institute
Kansas City, Missouri

Pierce J. Vatterott, MD, FACC
Co-Director of Arrhythmia Center
St. Paul Heart Clinic
St. Paul, Minnesota

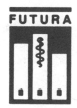

FUTURA

Futura Publishing
Company, Inc.
Armonk, NY

Library of Congress Cataloging-in-Publication Data
ECG board review and study guide : criteria definitions / by James H. O'Keefe, Jr. ... [et al.].
    p.   cm.
  ISBN 0-87993-600-2
  1. Electrocardiography—Examinations, questions, etc.
I. O'Keefe, Jr., James H.
  [DNLM: 1. Electrocardiography—examination questions.   2. Heart Diseases—diagnosis—examination
questions.   WG 18 E17 1994]
RC683.5.E5E24   1994
616.1'207547'076—dc20
DNLM/DLC
for Library of Congress   94-29343
                                                                                                          CIP

Copyright 1994
Futura Publishing Company, Inc.

Published by
Futura Publishing Company, Inc.
135 Bedford Road
Armonk, New York 10504

LC #: 94-29343
ISBN #: 087993-600-2

Every effort has been made to ensure that the information in this book is as up to date and as accurate as possible at the time of publication. However, due to the constant developments in medicine, neither the author, nor the editor, nor the publisher can accept any legal or any other responsibility for any errors or omissions that may occur.

Printed in the United States of America on acid-free paper.

Contents

Sample ECGs

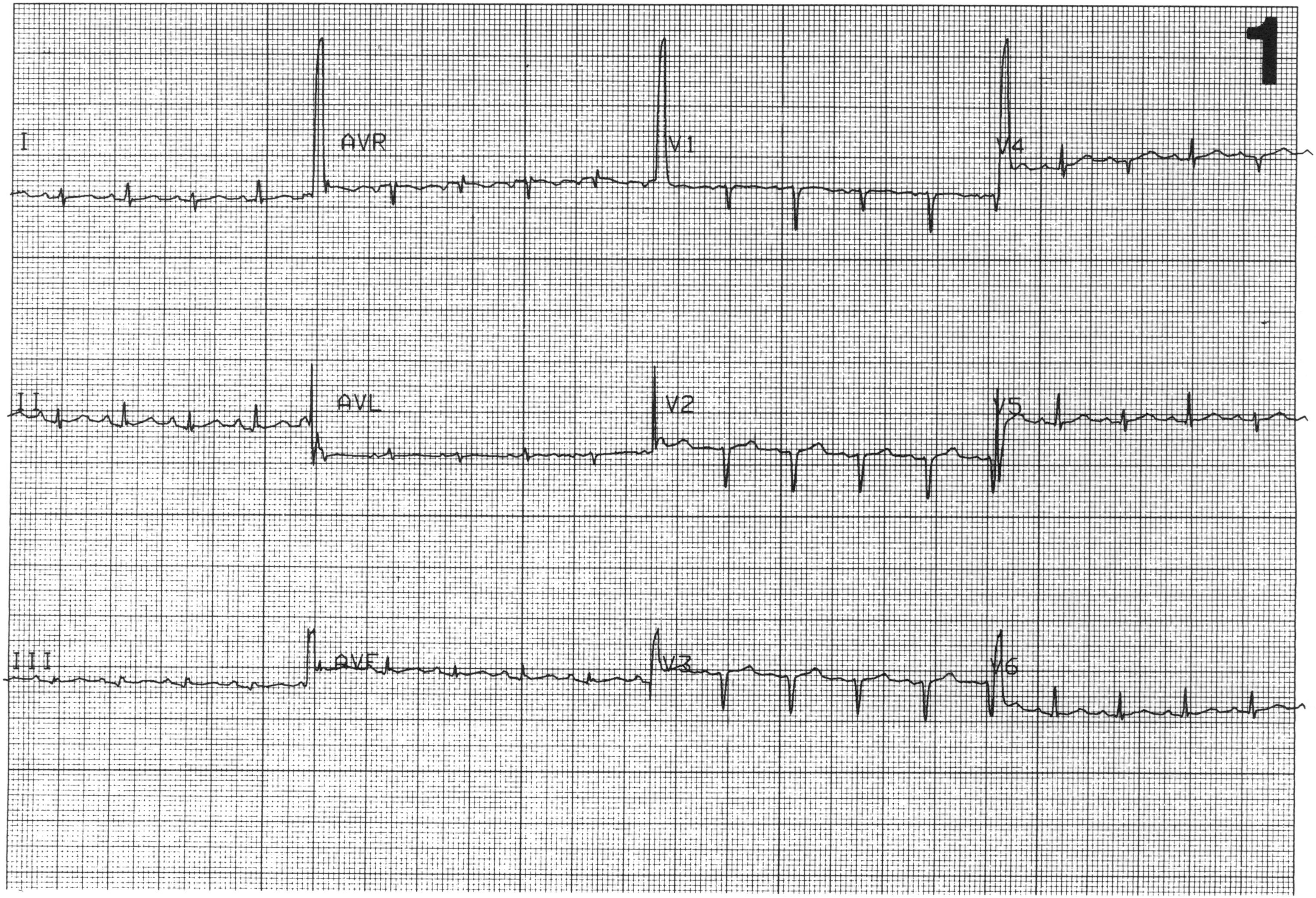
1
I
AVR
V1
V4
II
AVL
V2
V5
III
AVF
V3
V6

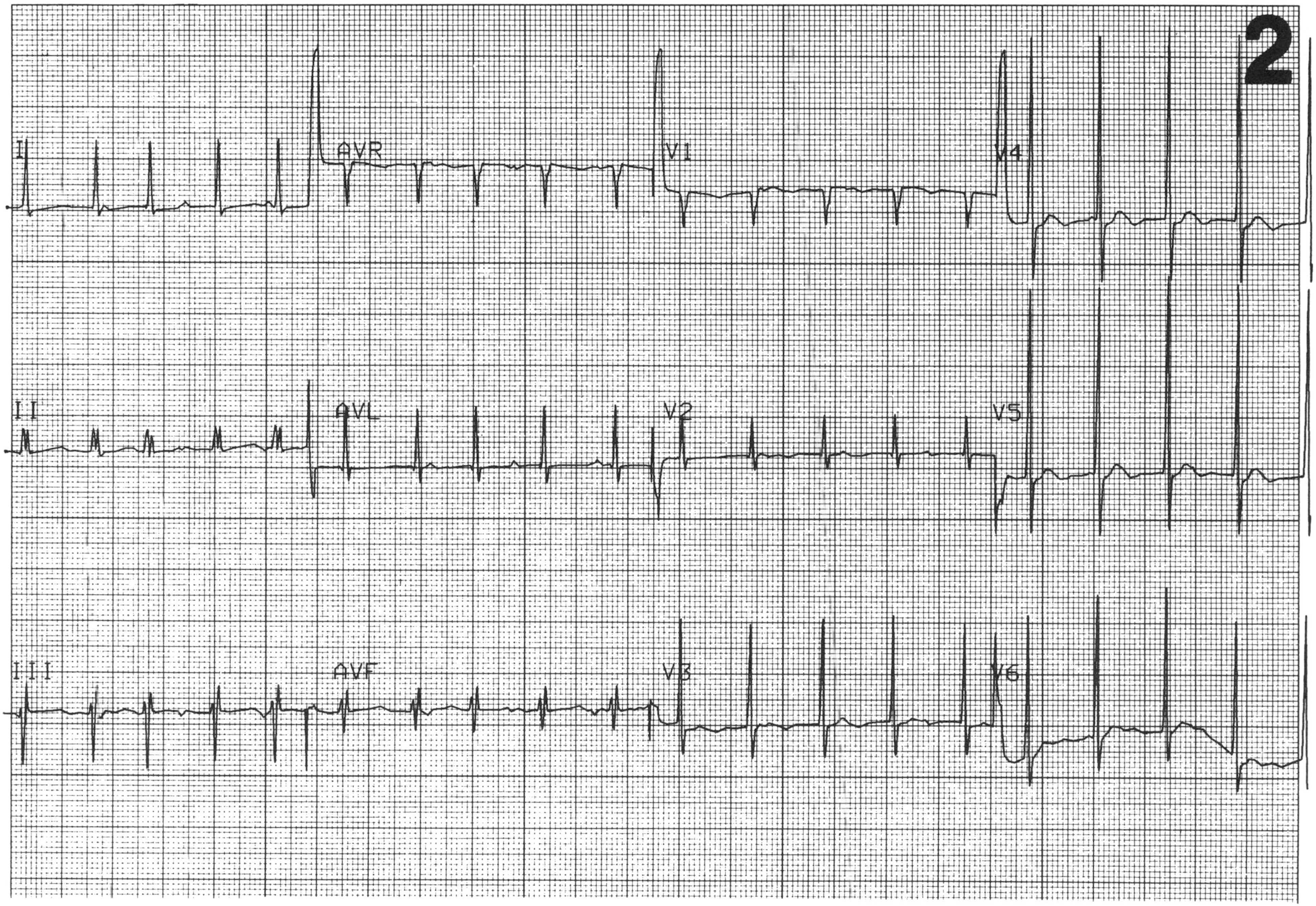
2
I
AVR
V1
V4
II
AVL
V2
V5
III
AVF
V3
V6

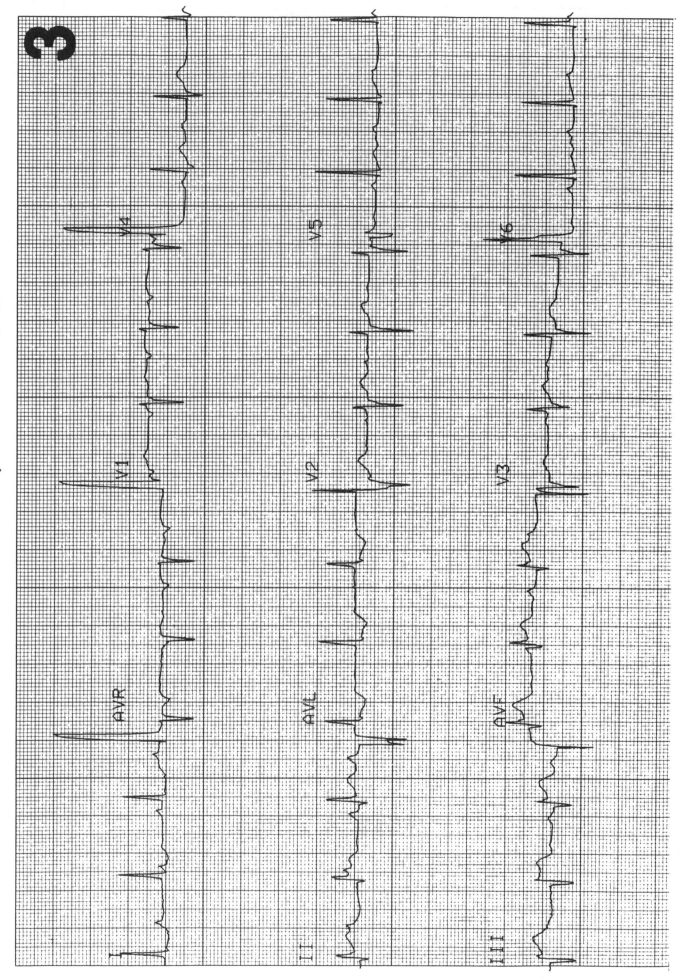

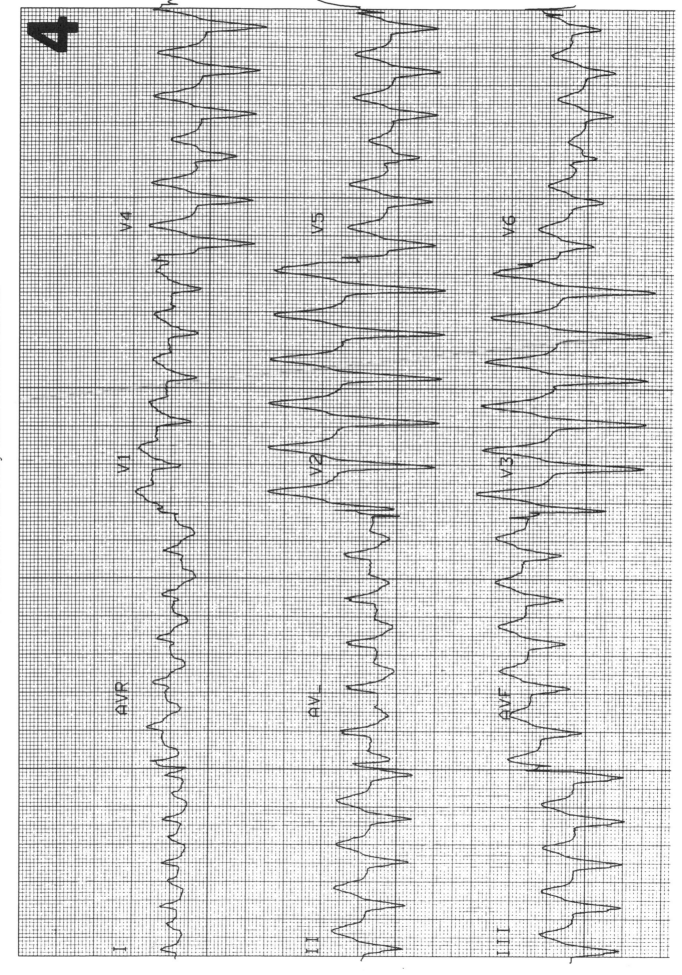

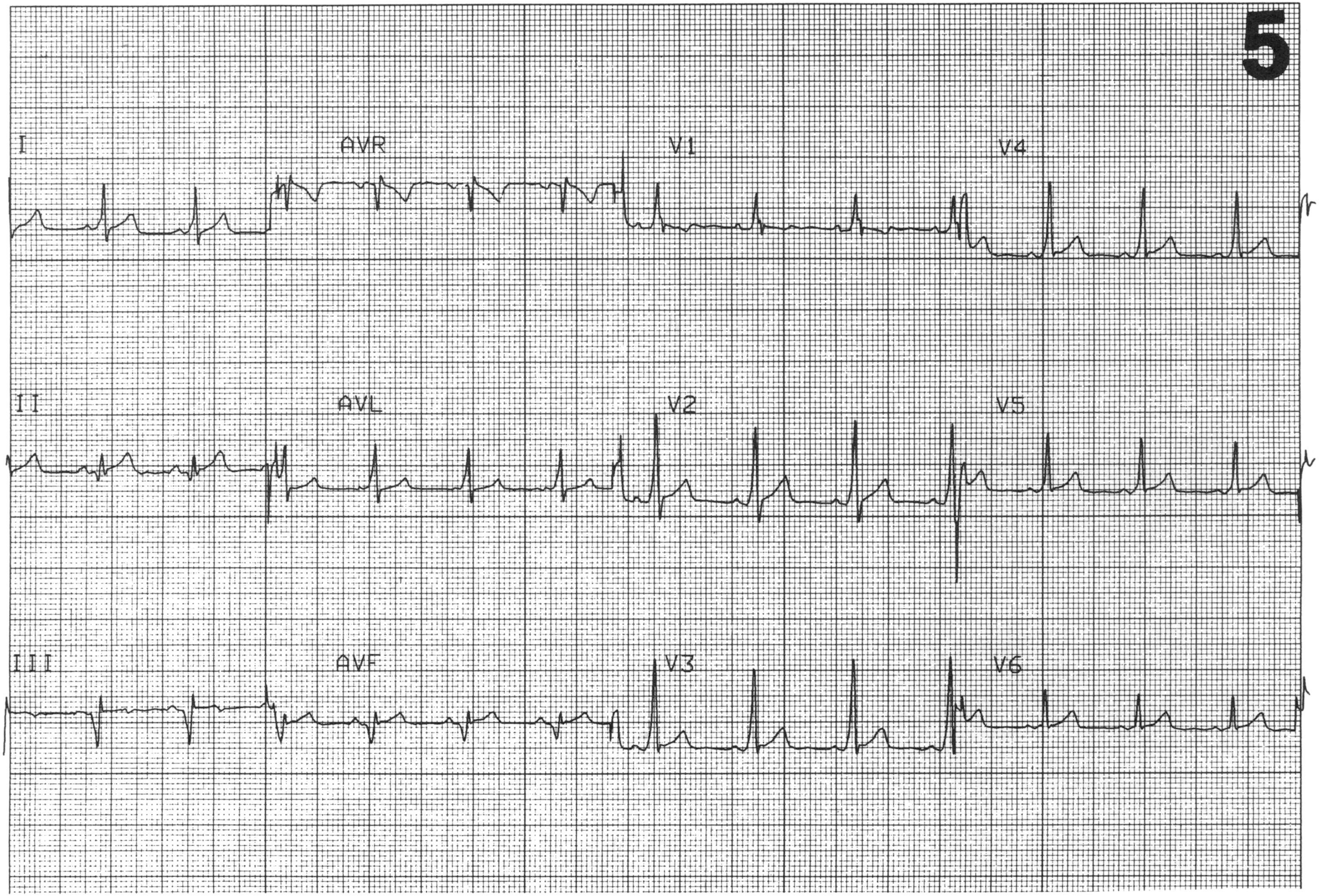
5
I
AVR
V1
V4
II
AVL
V2
V5
III
AVF
V3
V6

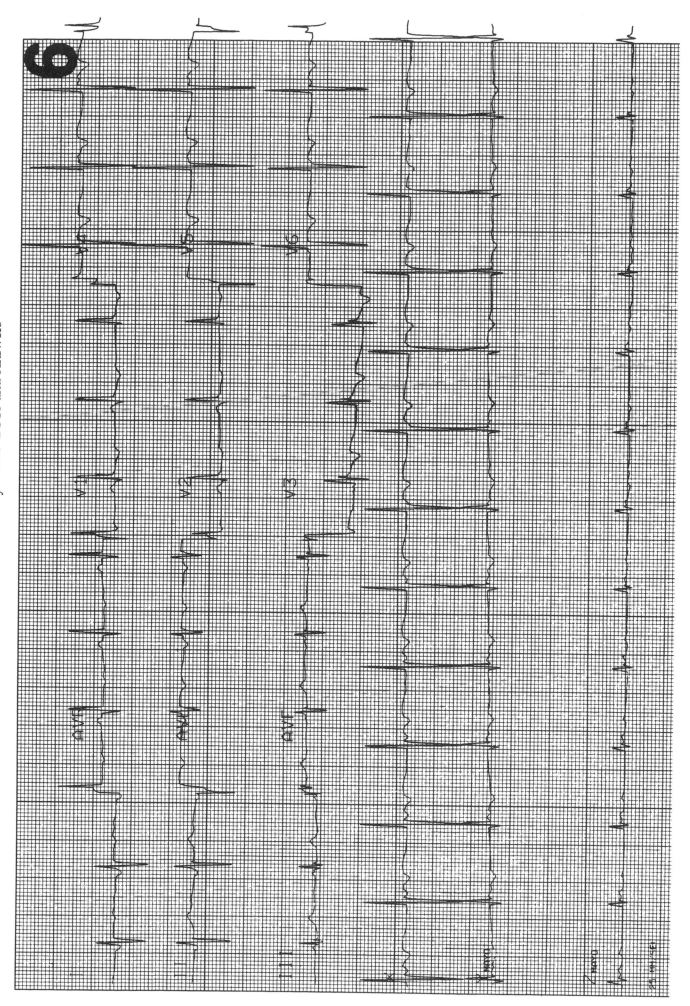

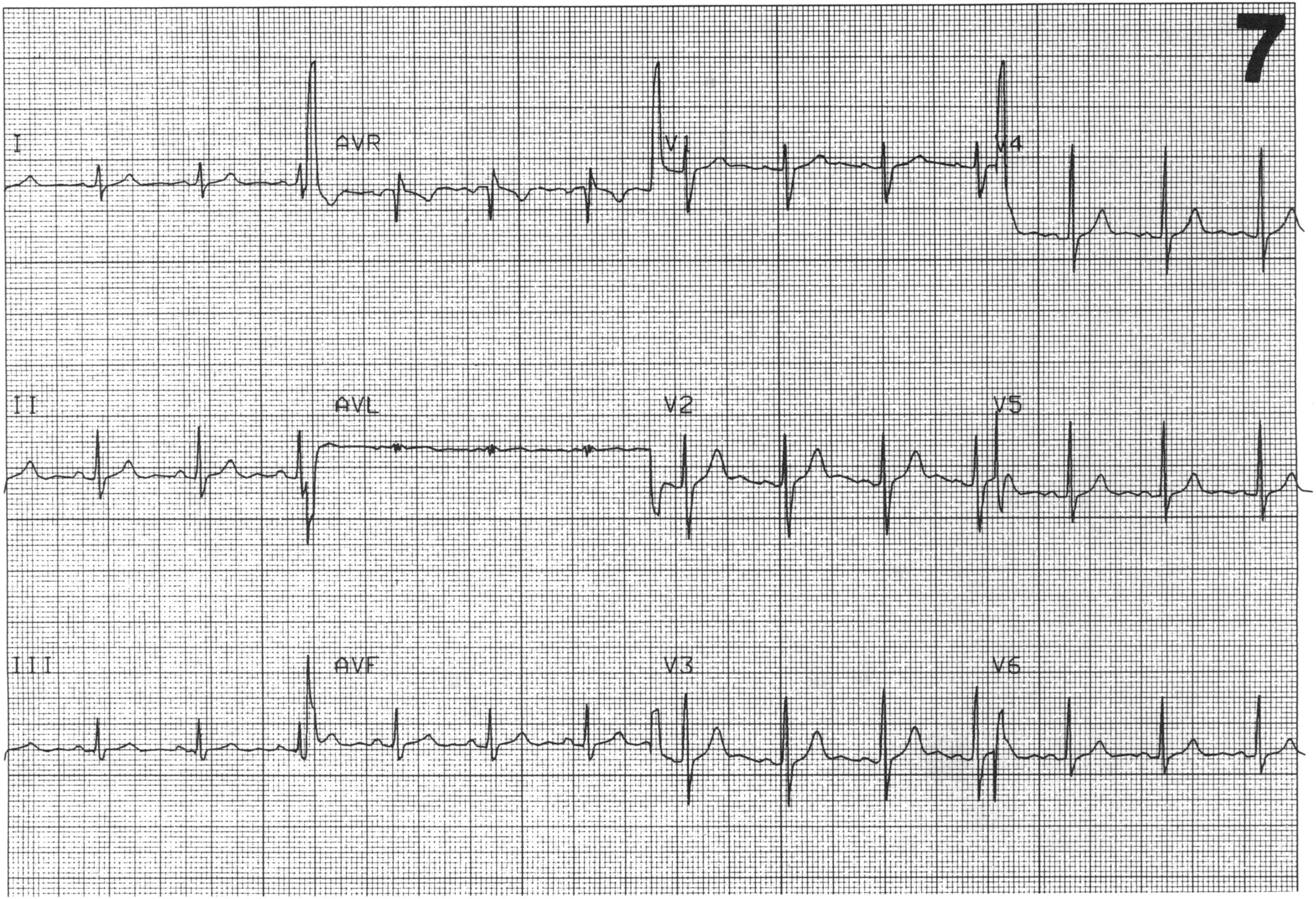
7
I
AVR
V1
V4
II
AVL
V2
V5
III
AVF
V3
V6

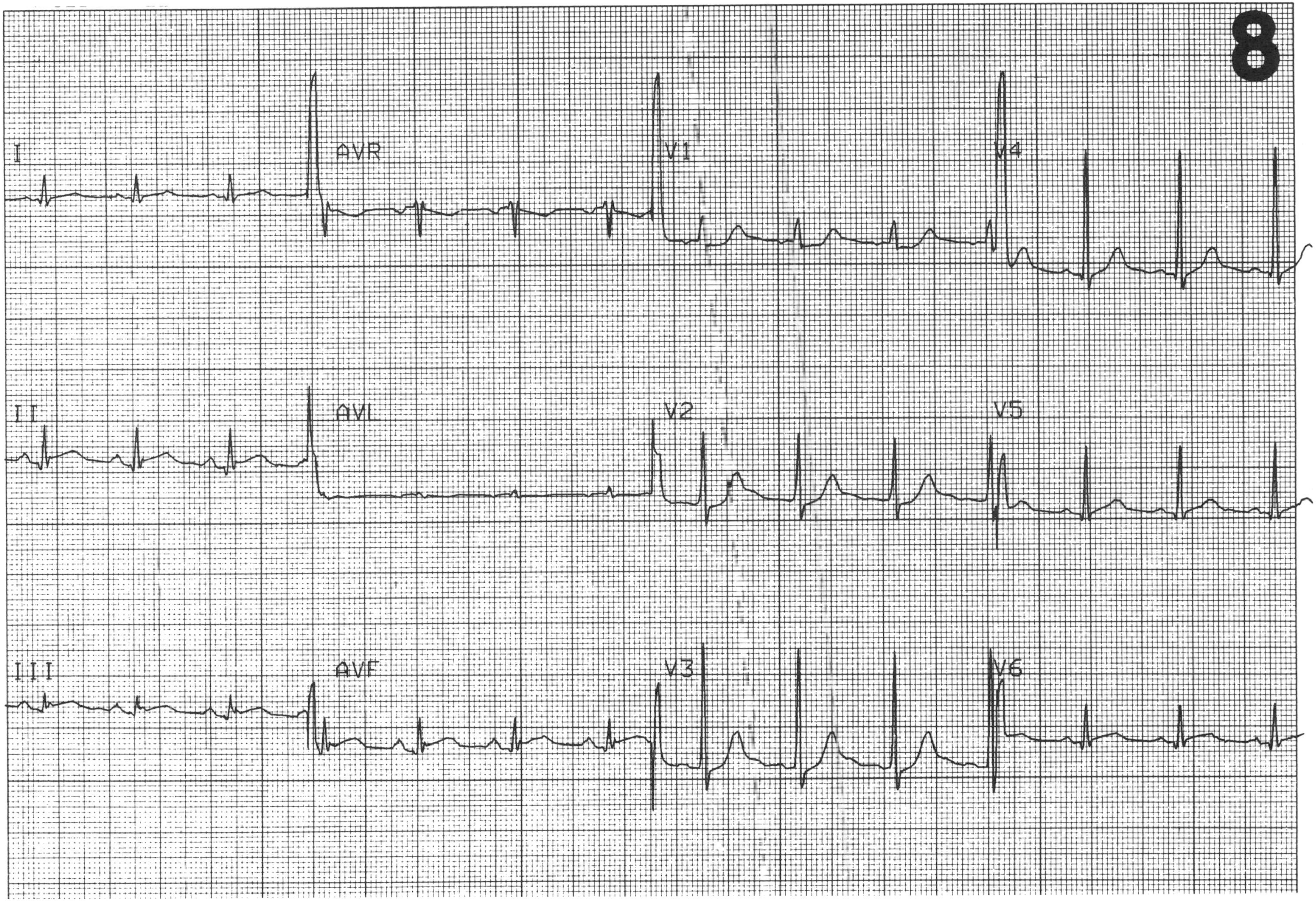
8
I
AVR
V1
V4
II
AVL
V2
V5
III
AVF
V3
V6

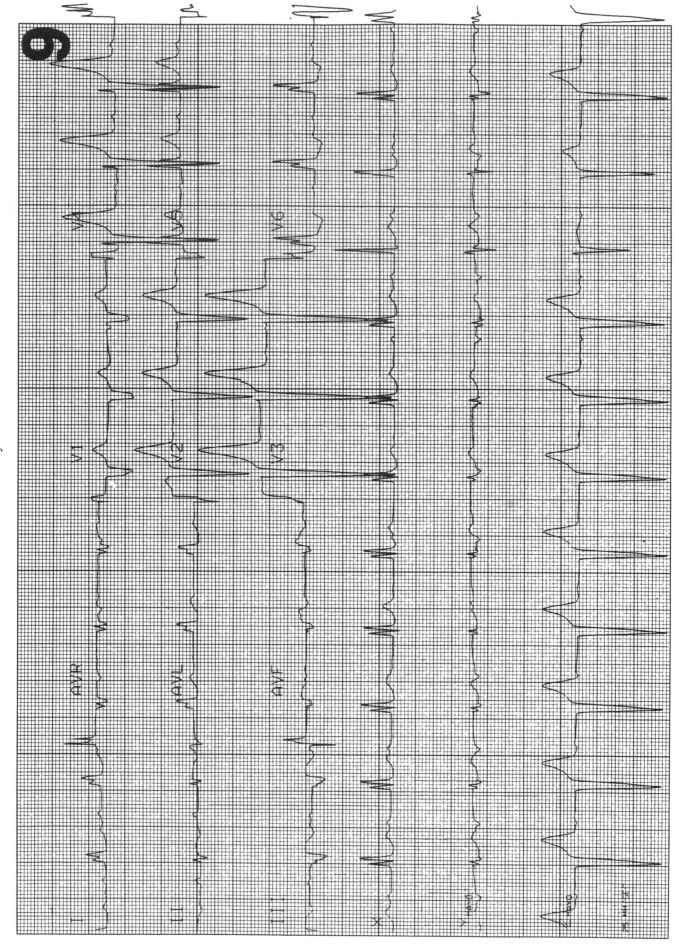

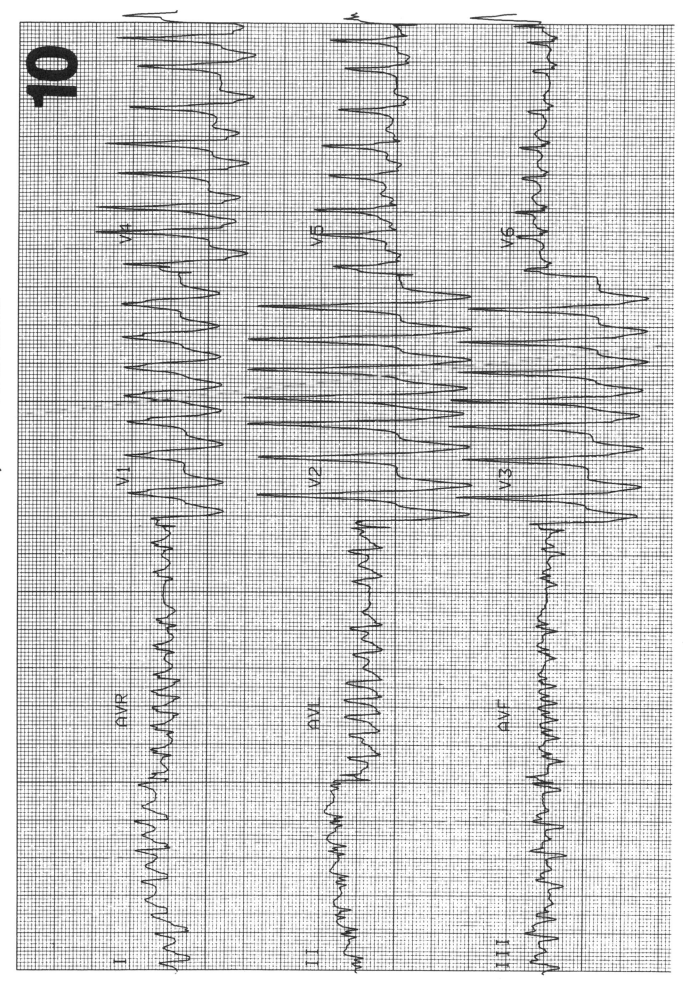

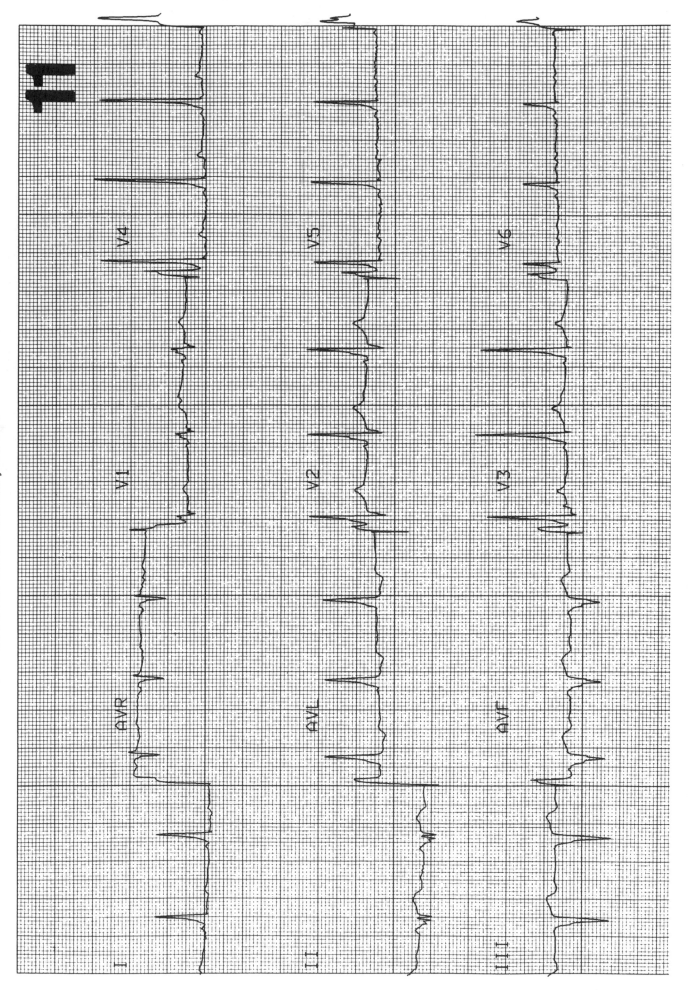

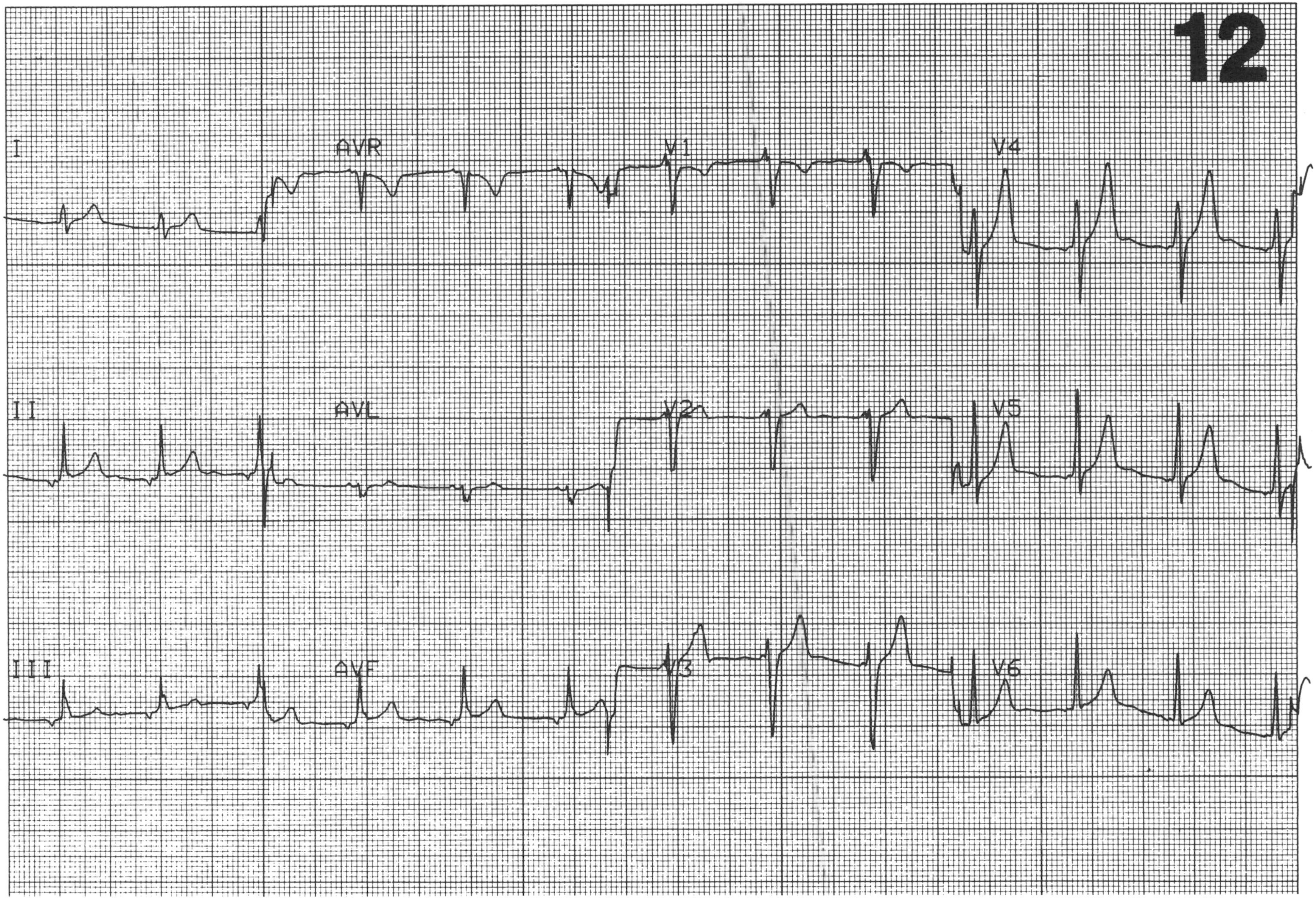
12
I
AVR
V1
V4
II
AVL
V2
V5
III
AVF
V3
V6

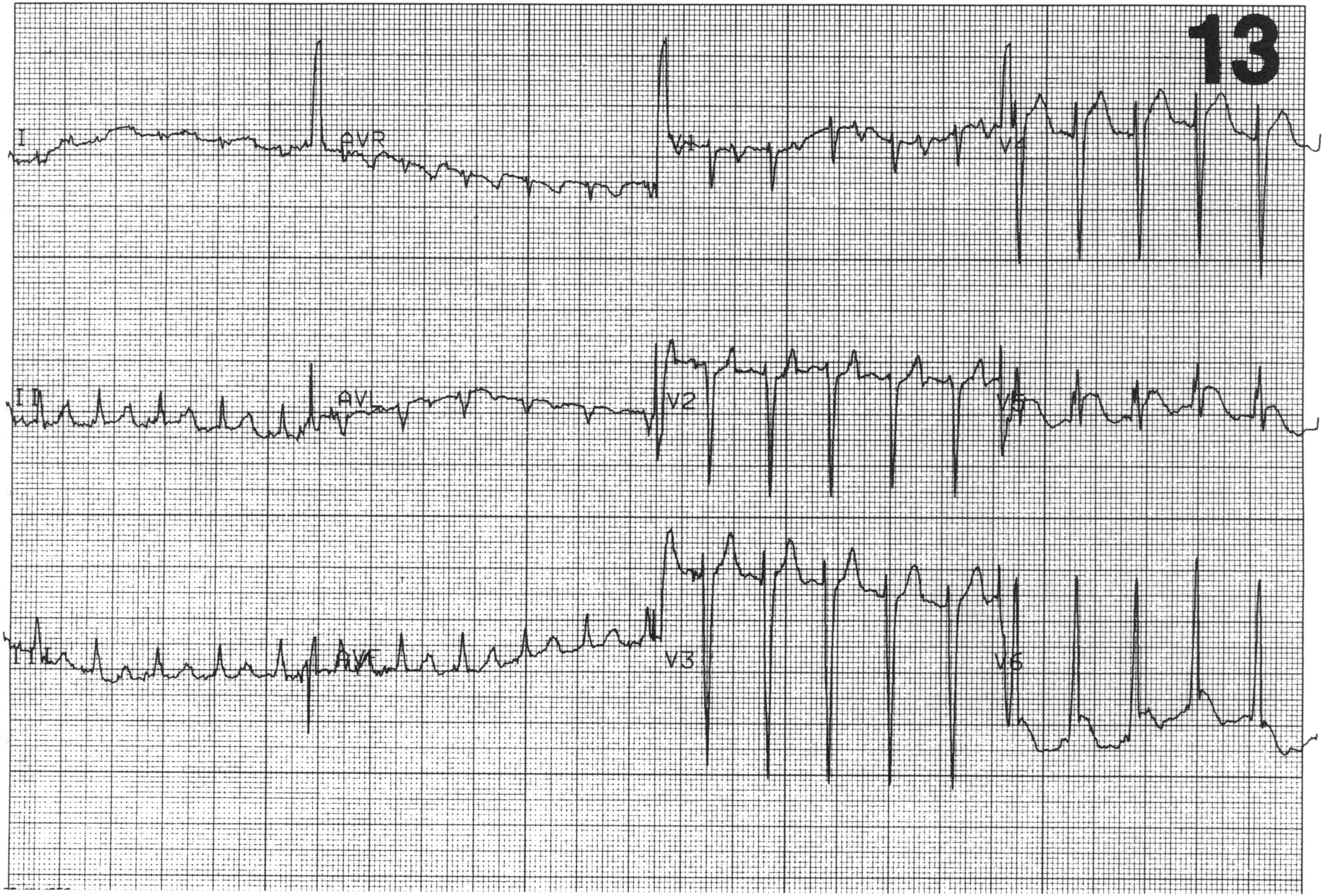
13
I
AVR
V1
V4
II
AVL
V2
V5
III
AVF
V3
V6

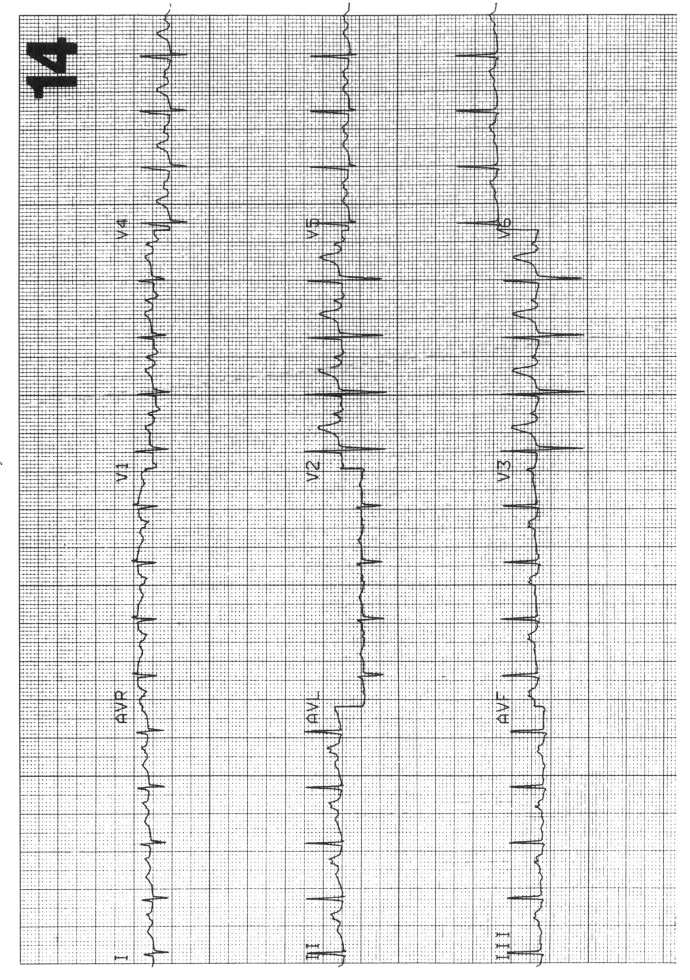

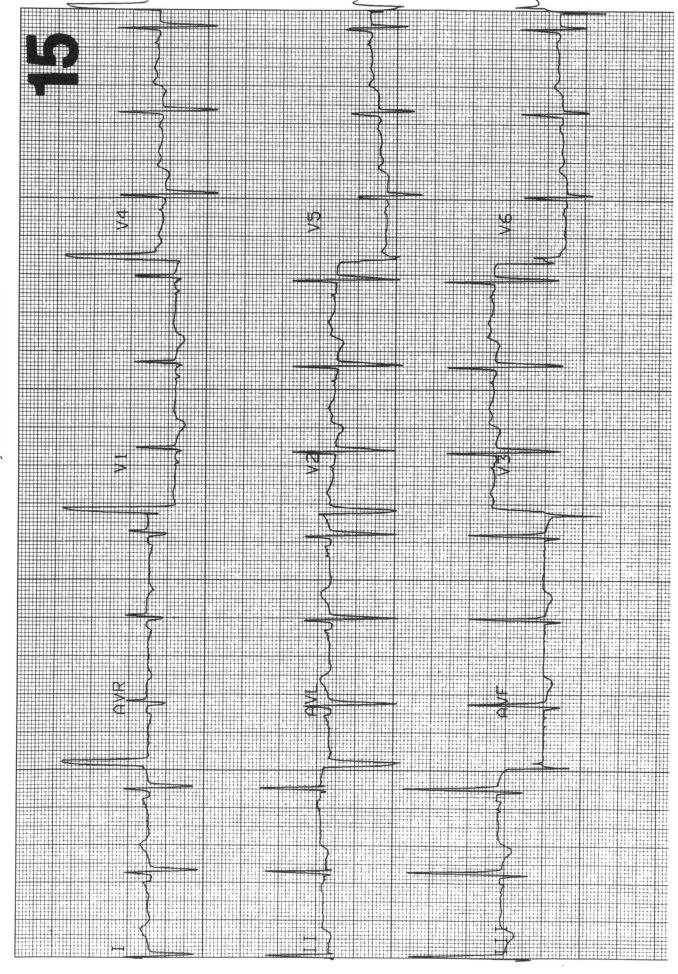

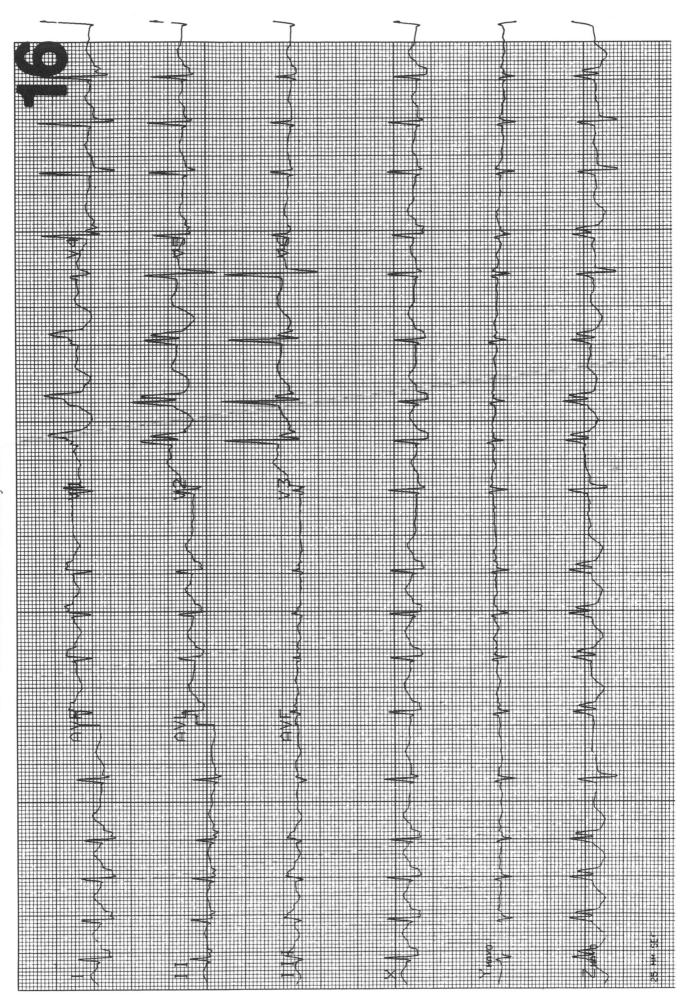

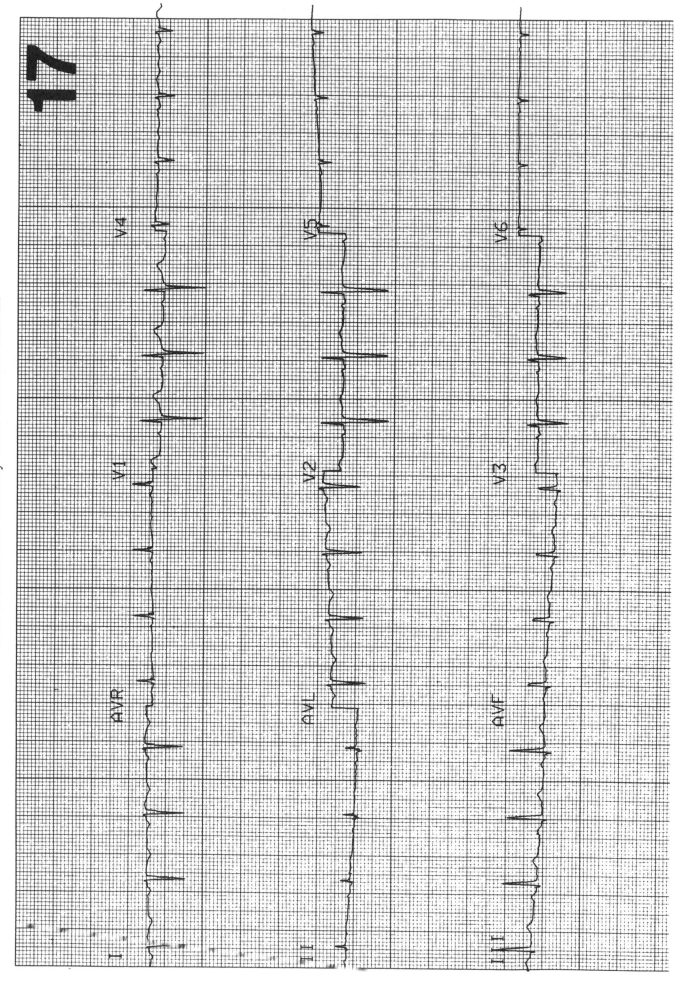

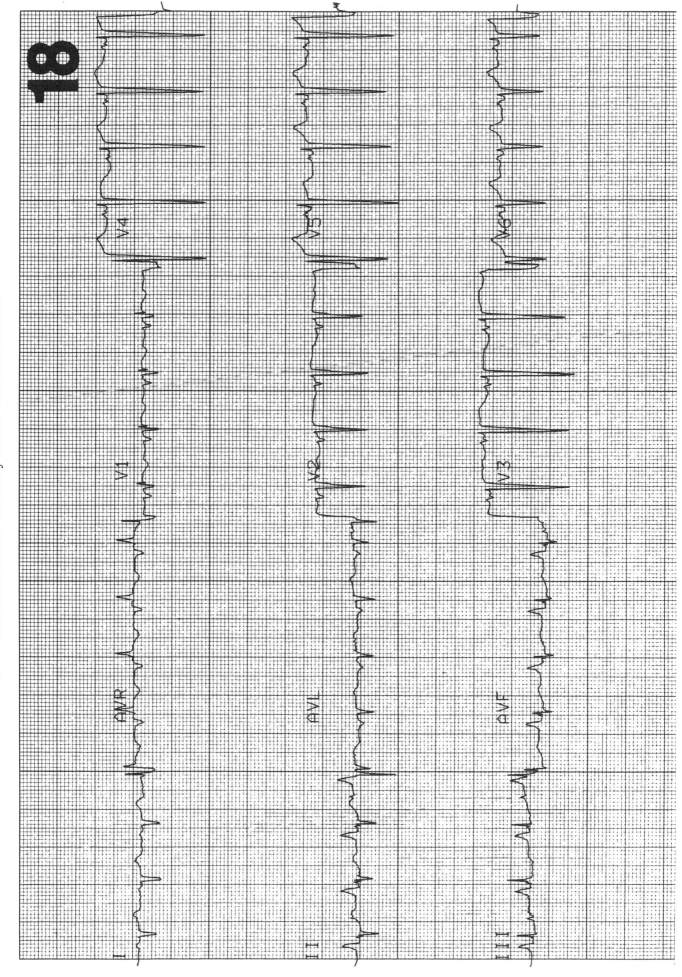

19

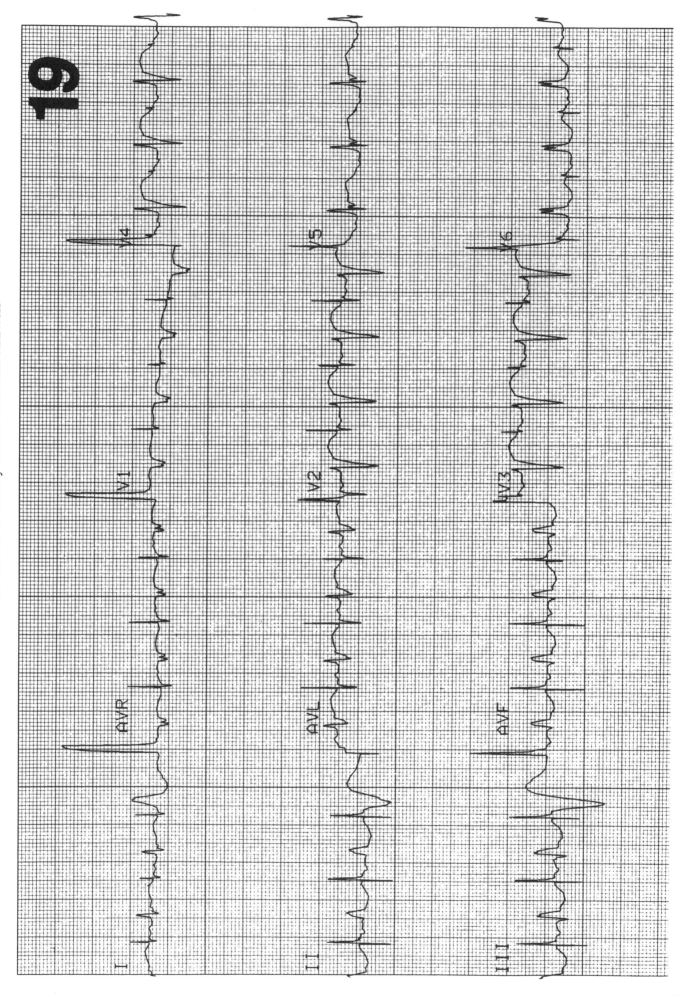

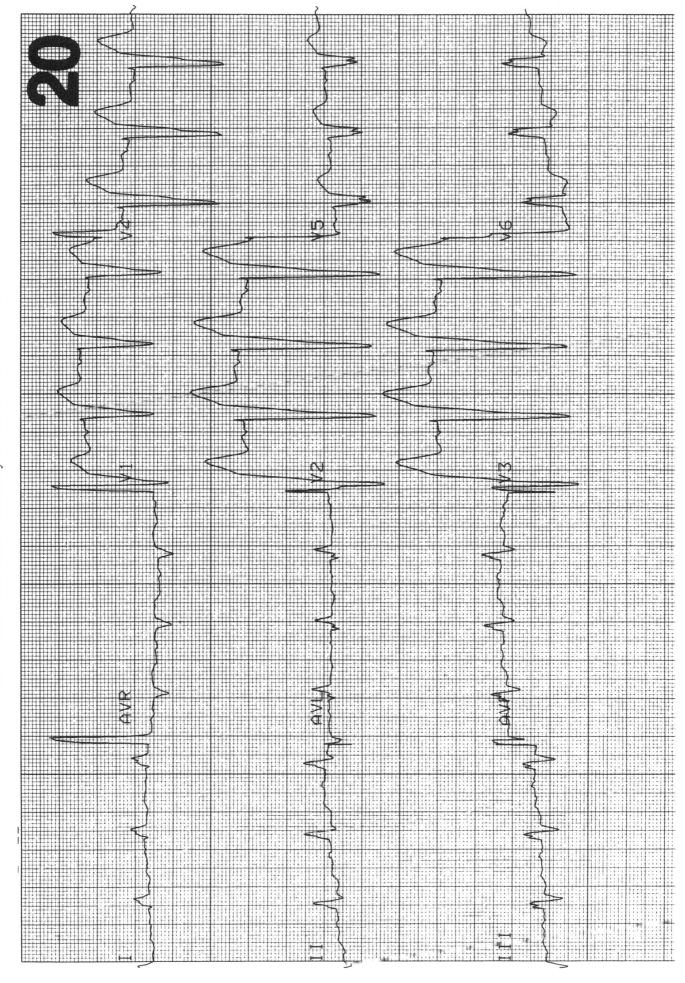

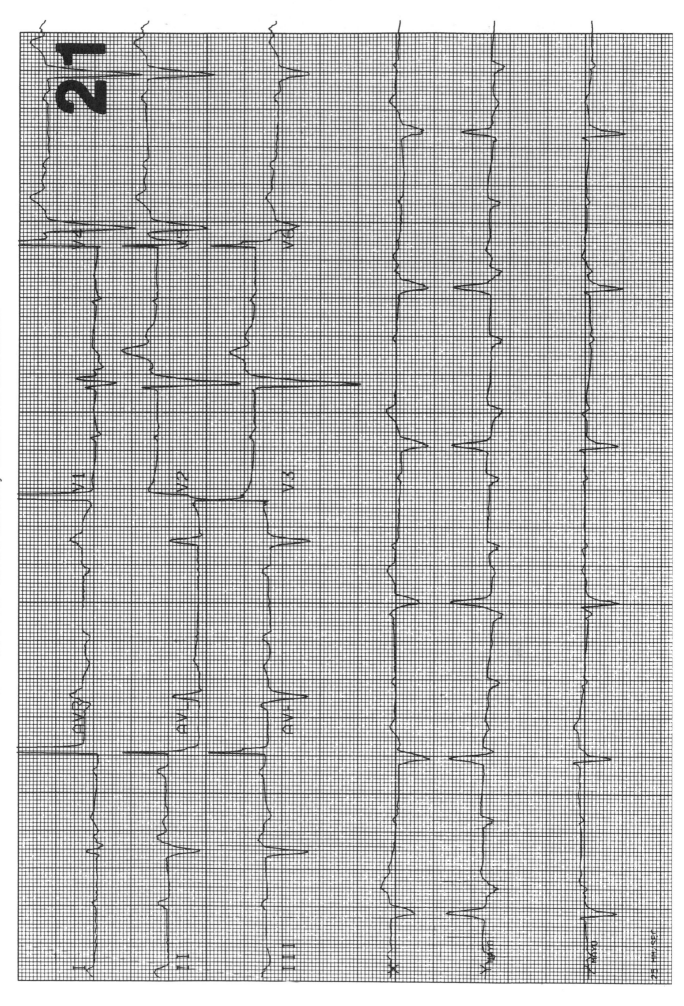

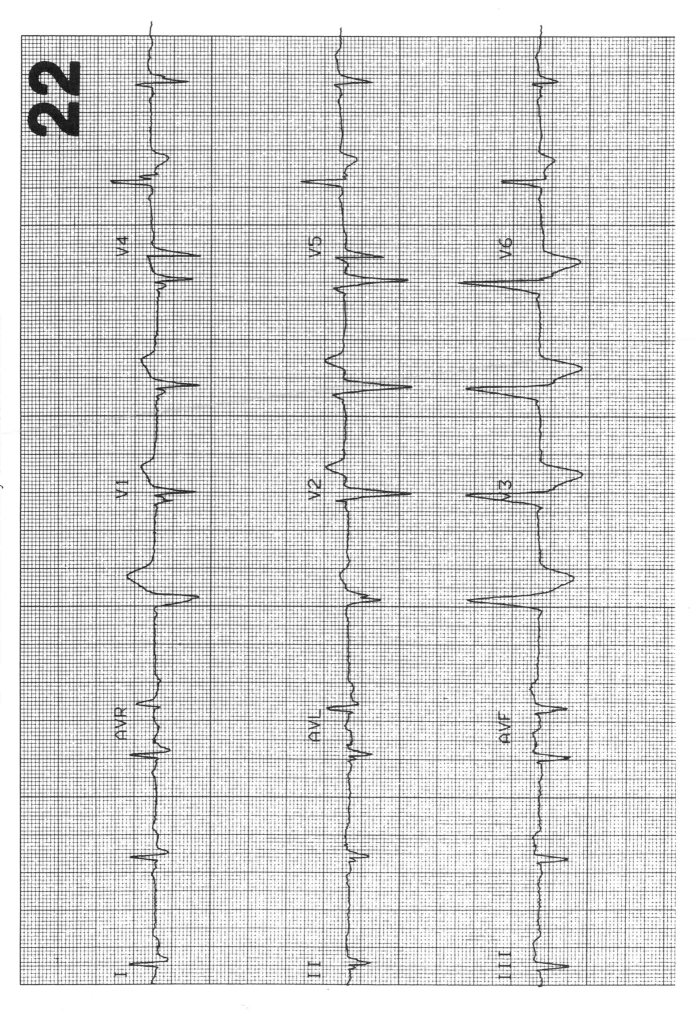

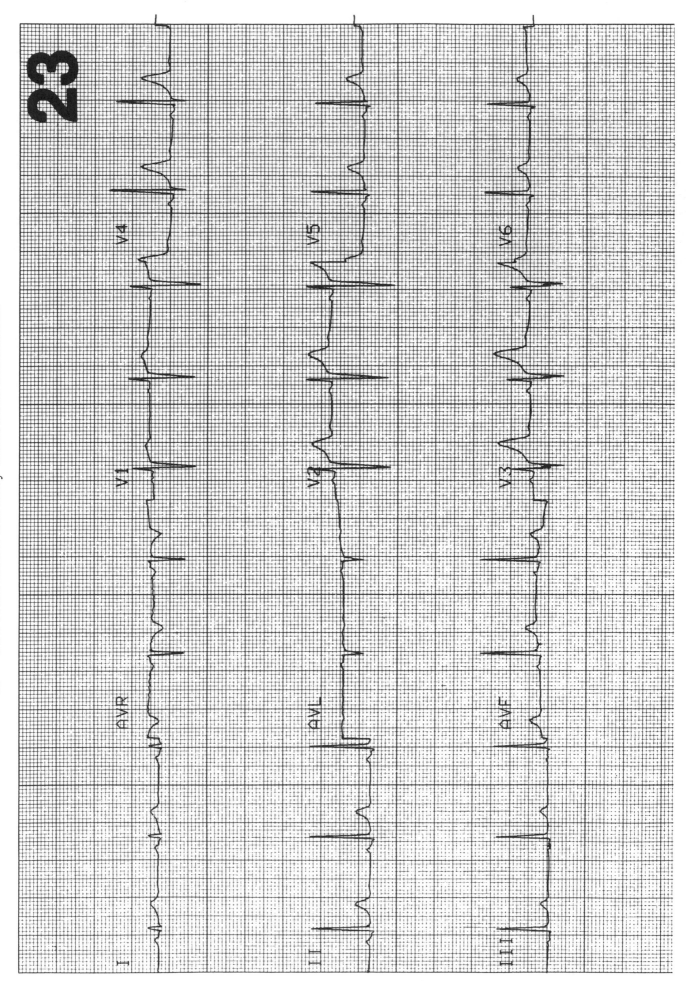

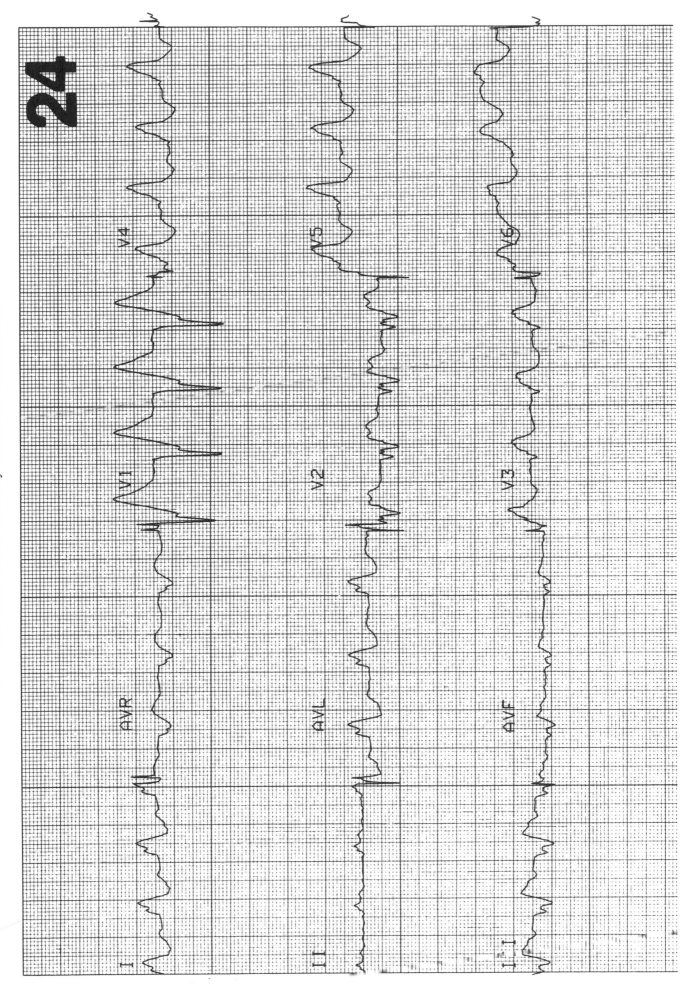

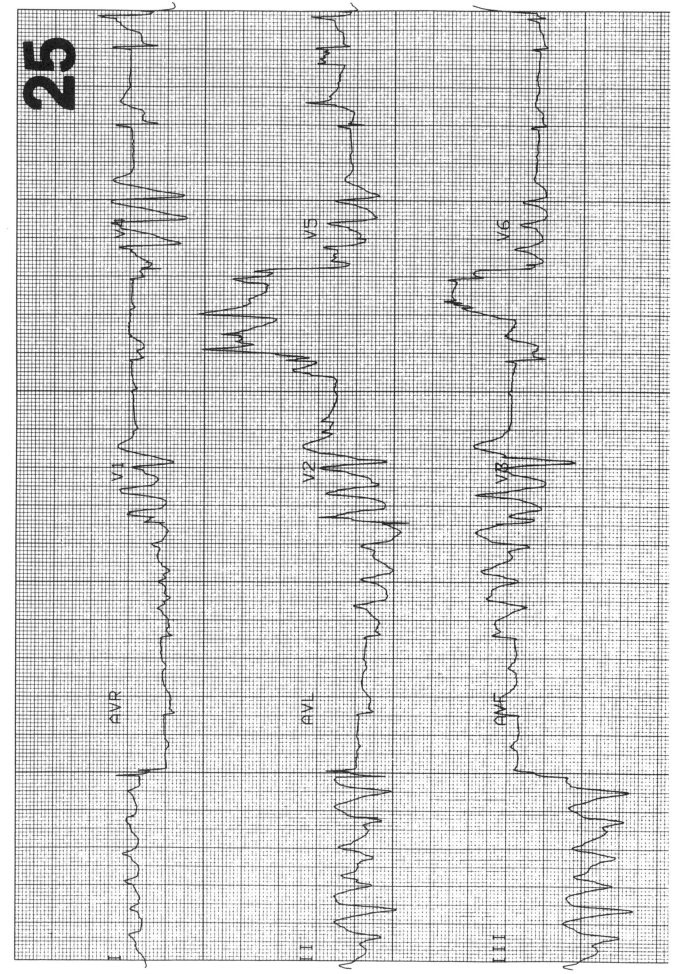

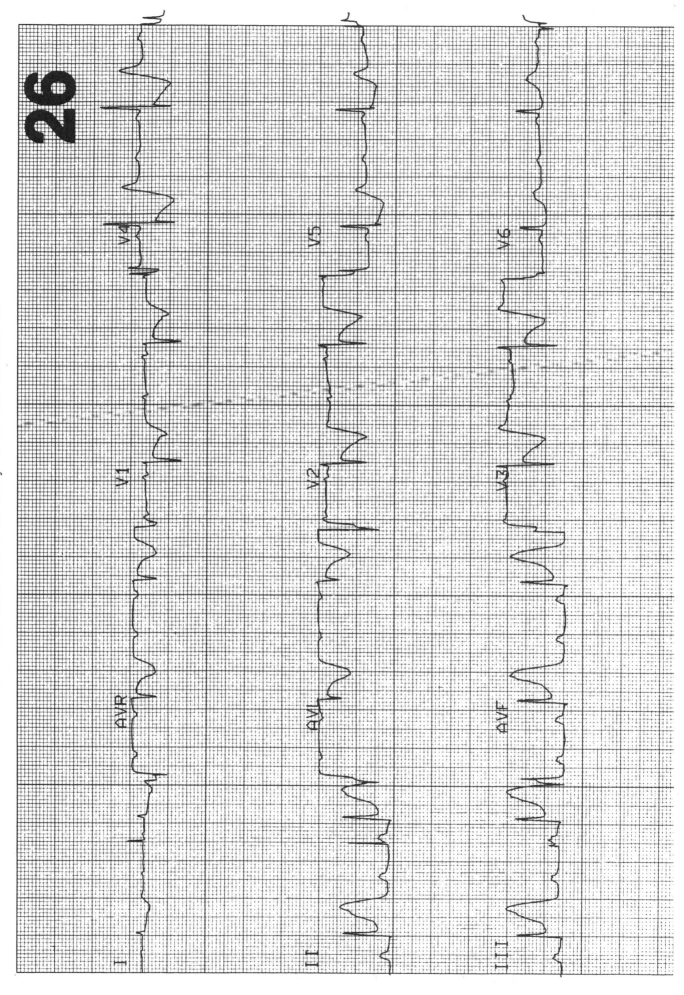

27

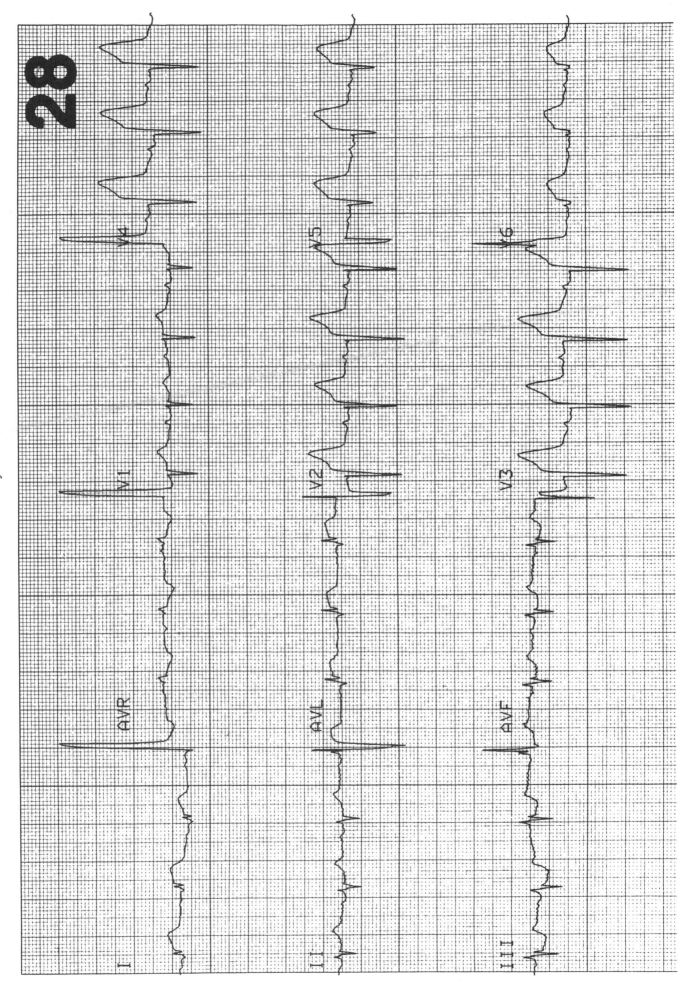

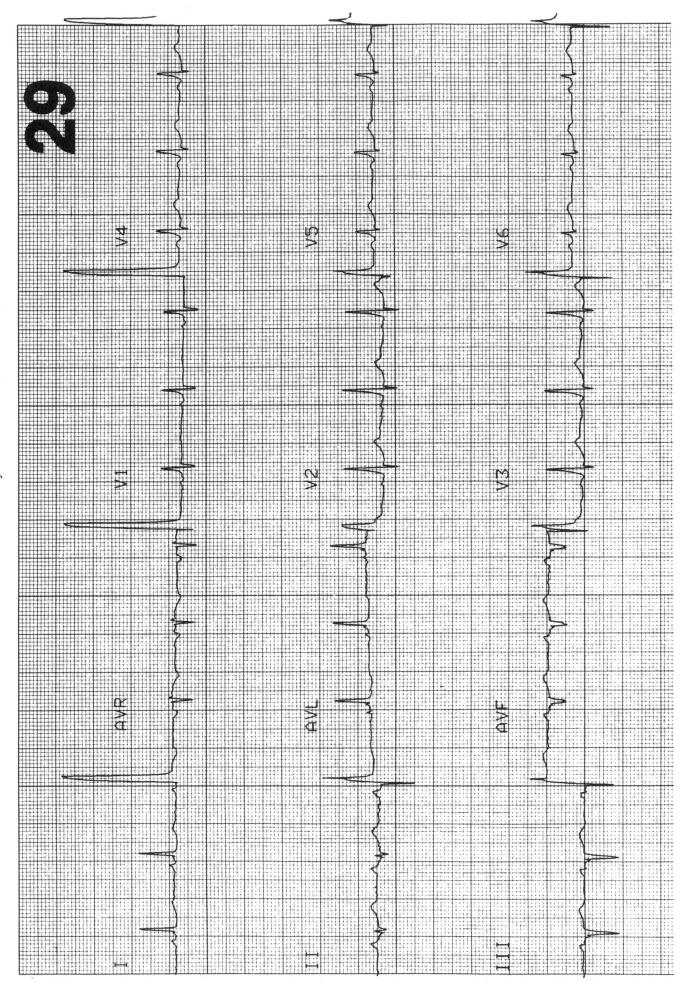

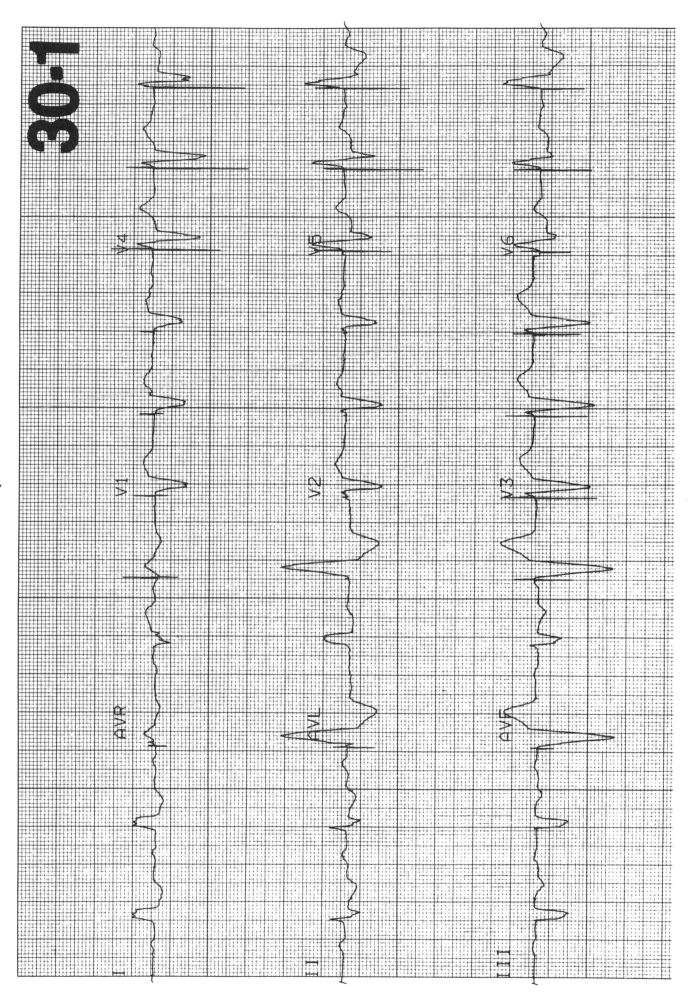

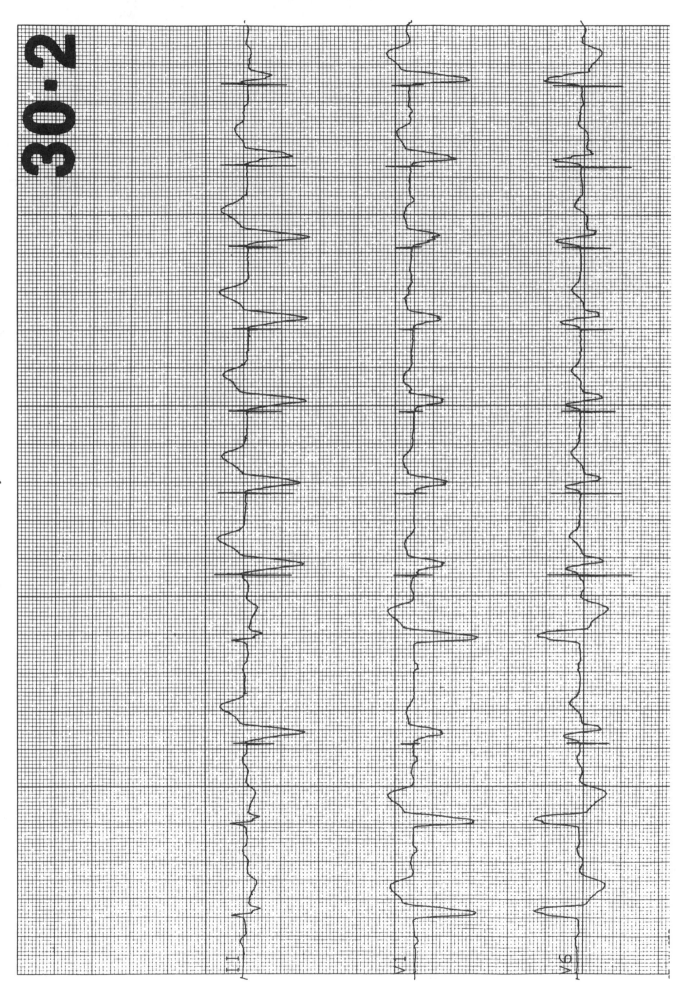

31

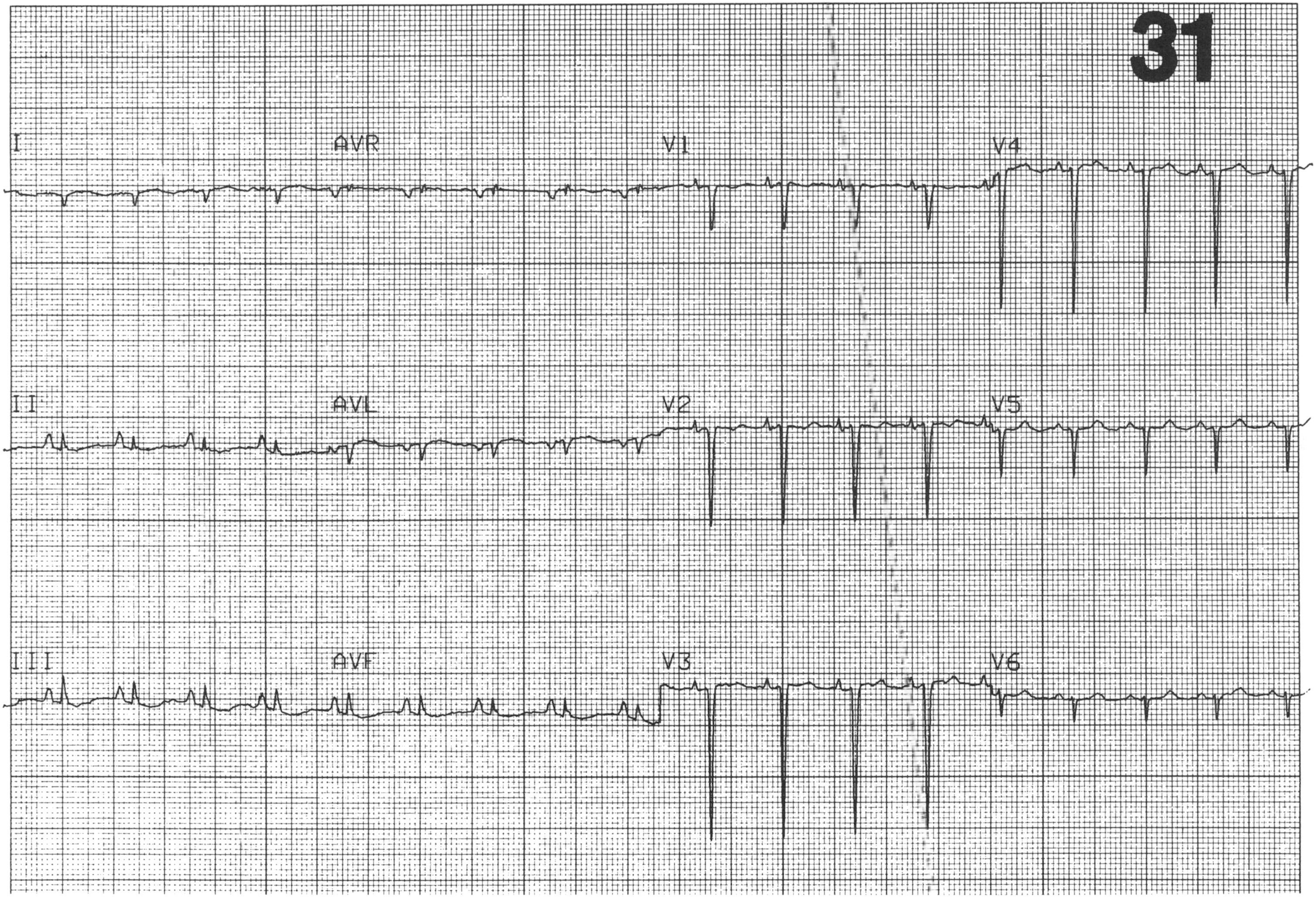

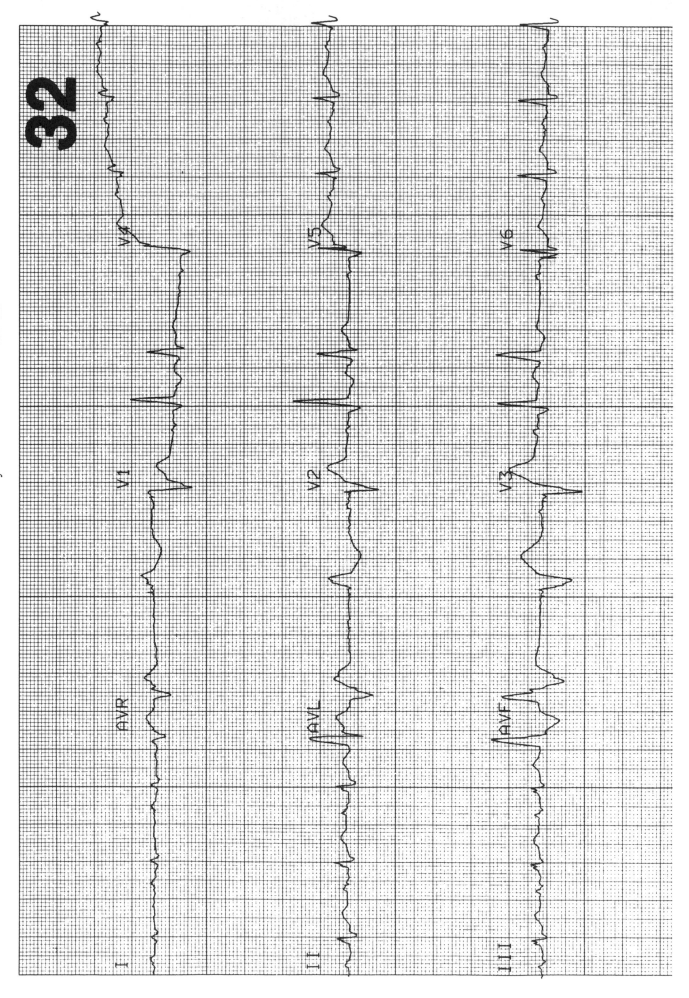

32

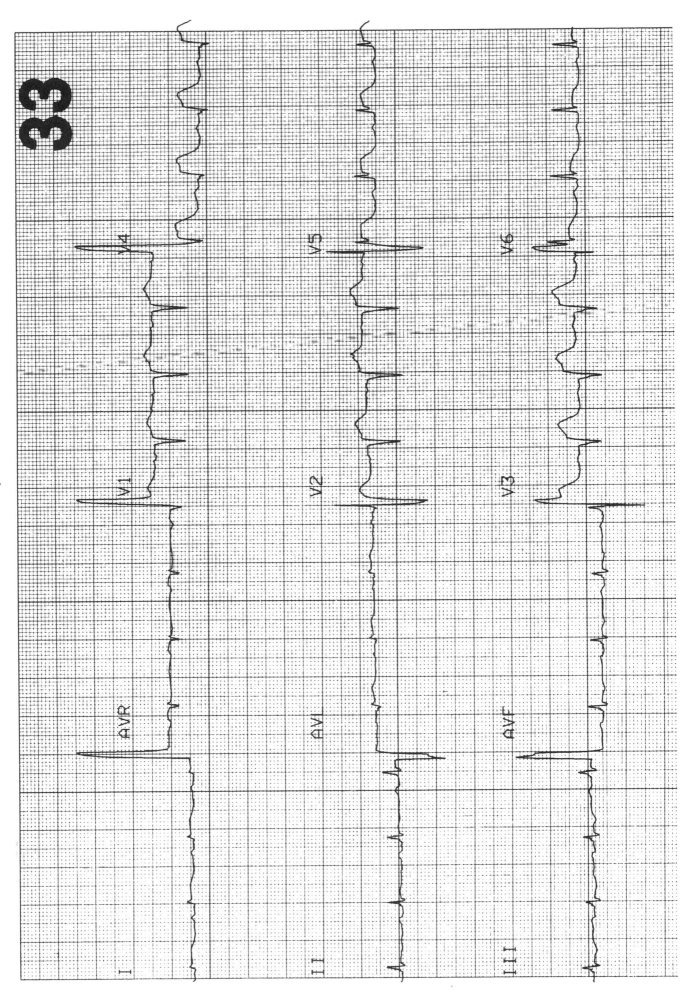

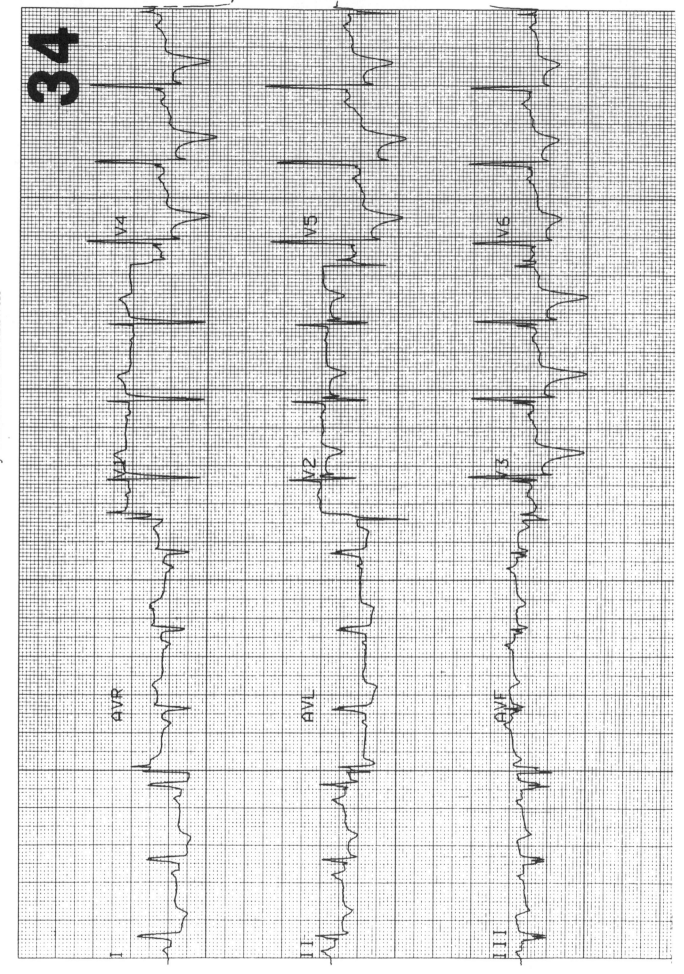

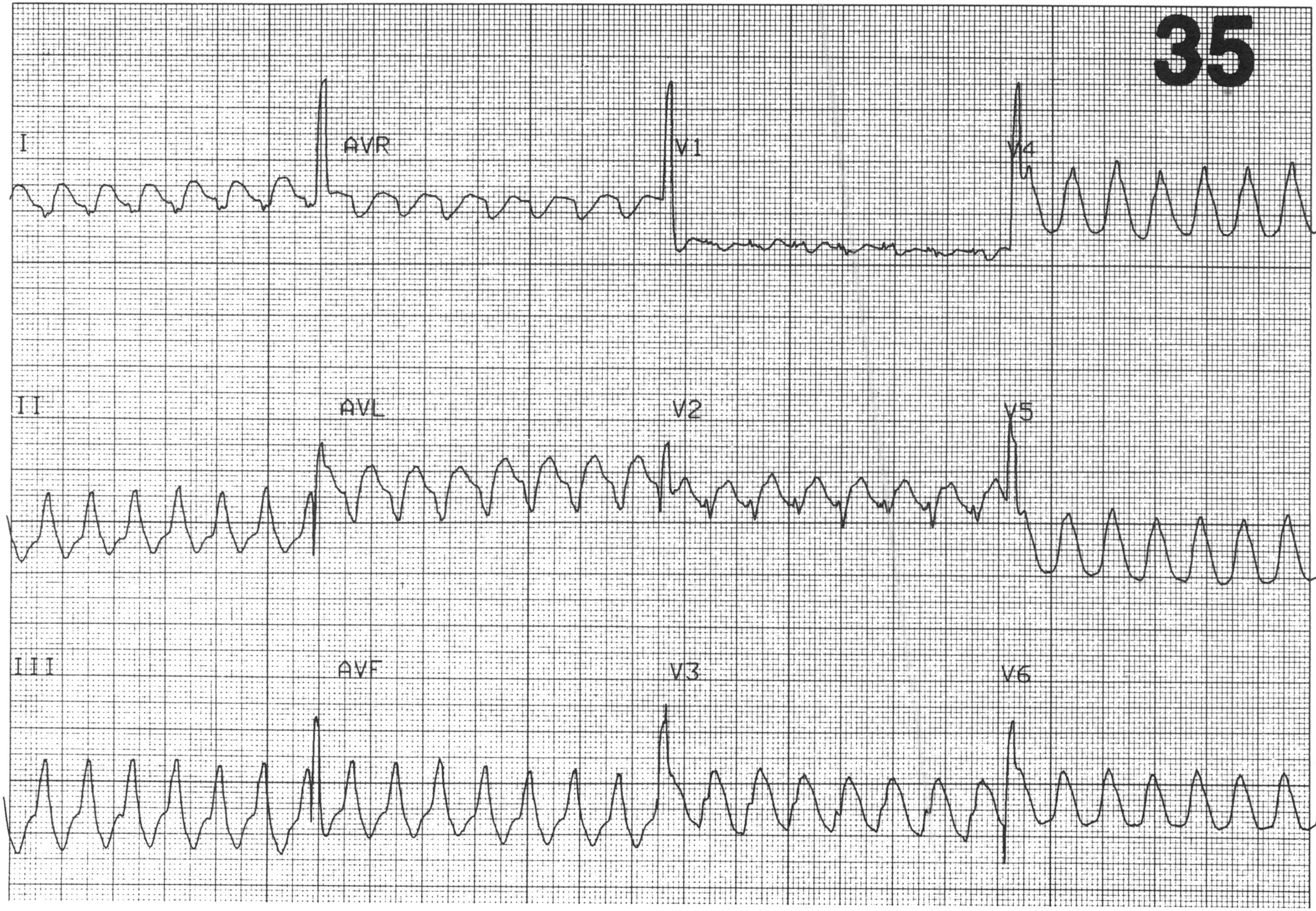
35
I
AVR
V1
V4
II
AVL
V2
V5
III
AVF
V3
V6

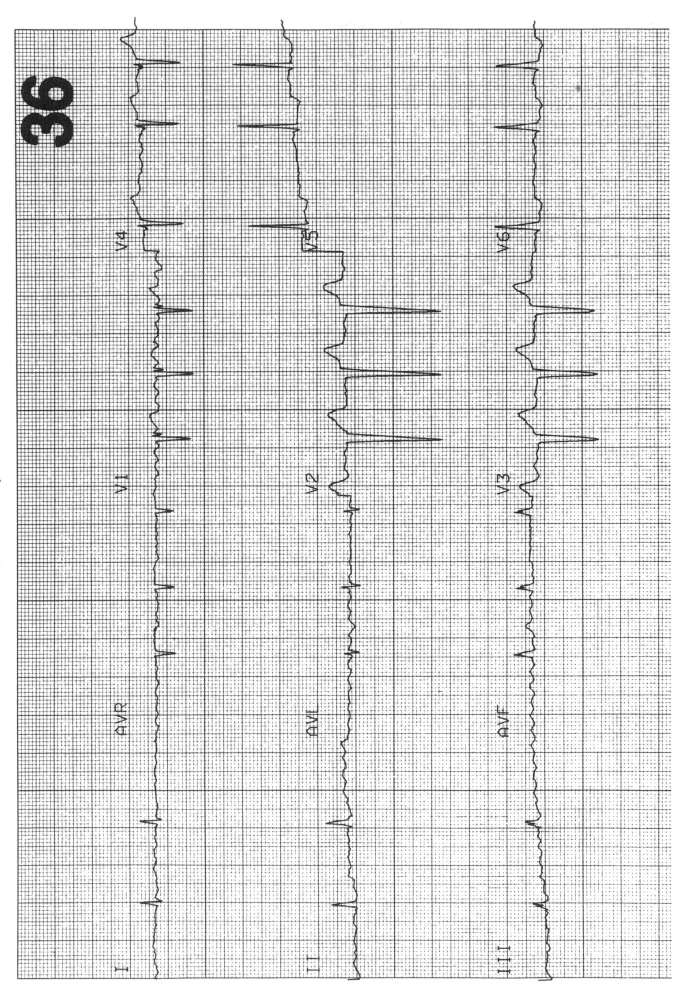

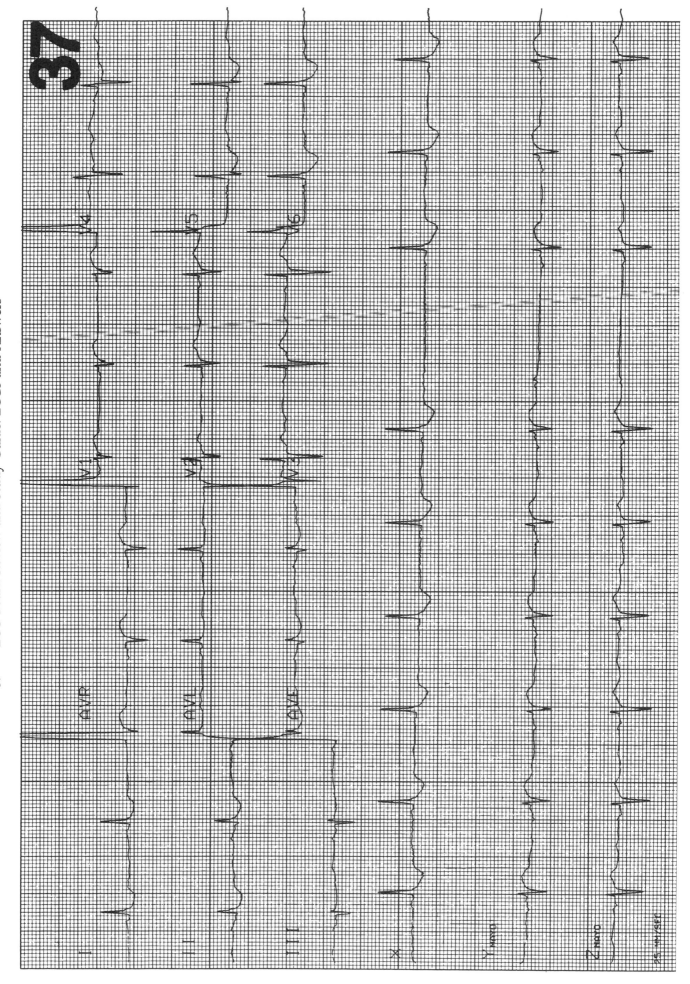

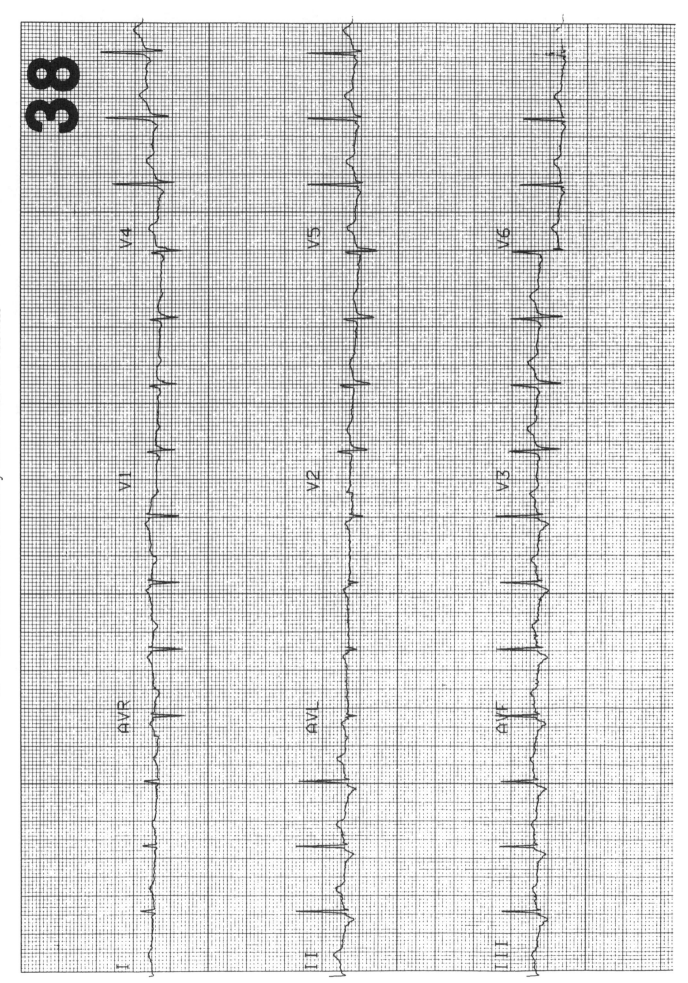

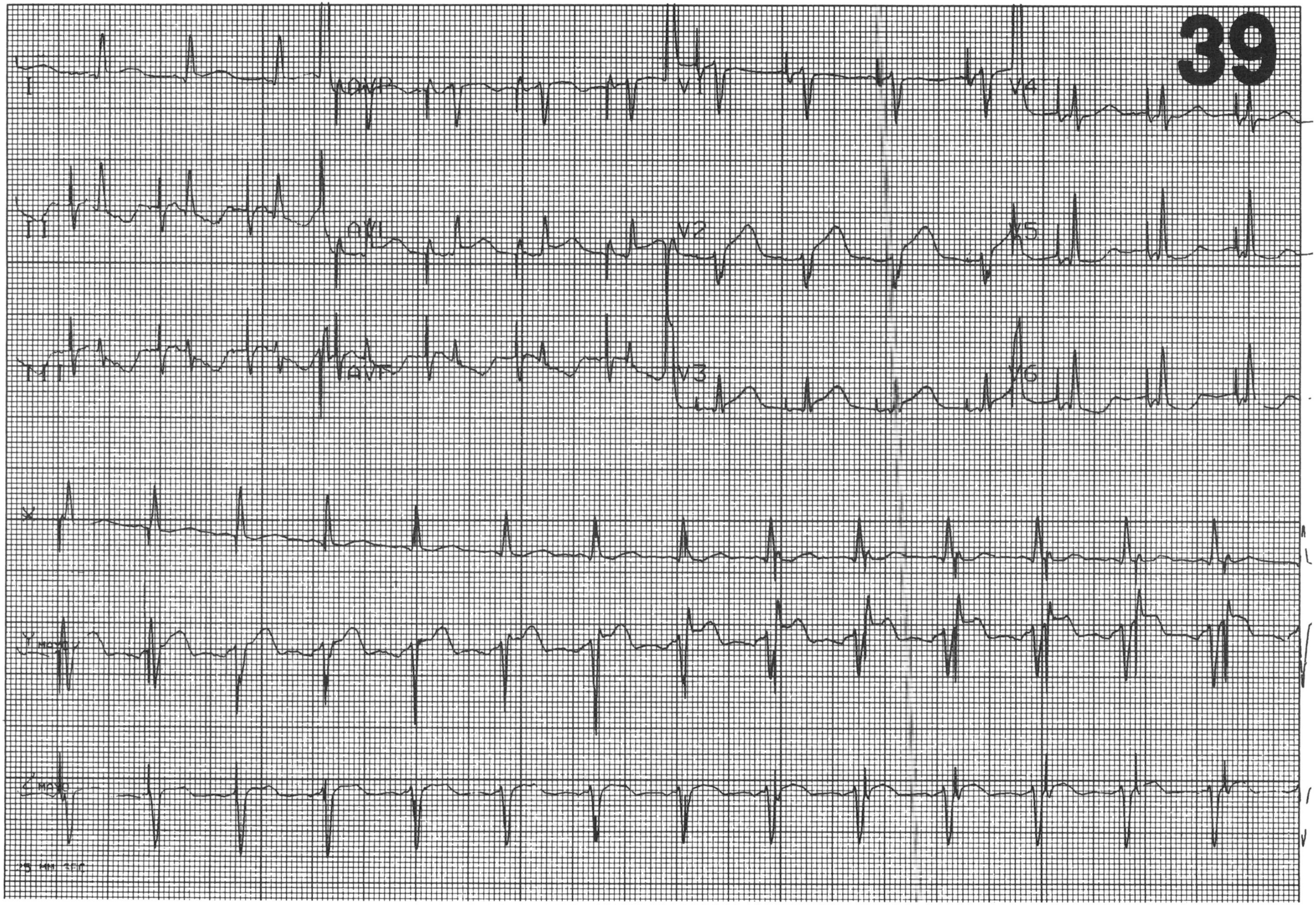
39
I
aVR
V1
V4
II
aVL
V2
V5
III
aVF
V3
V6
X
Y
Z

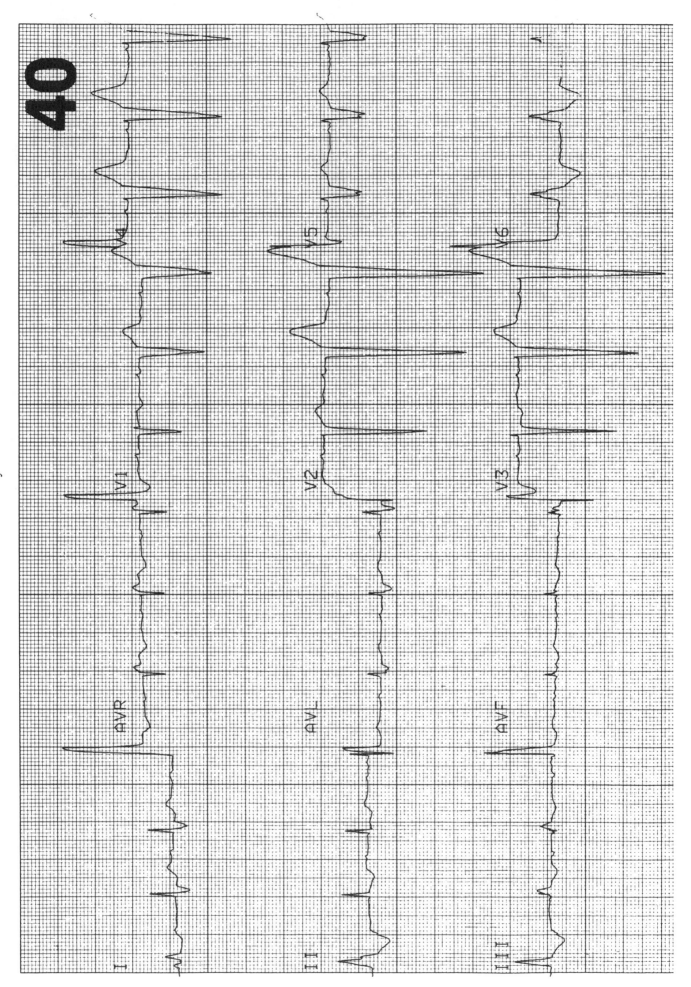

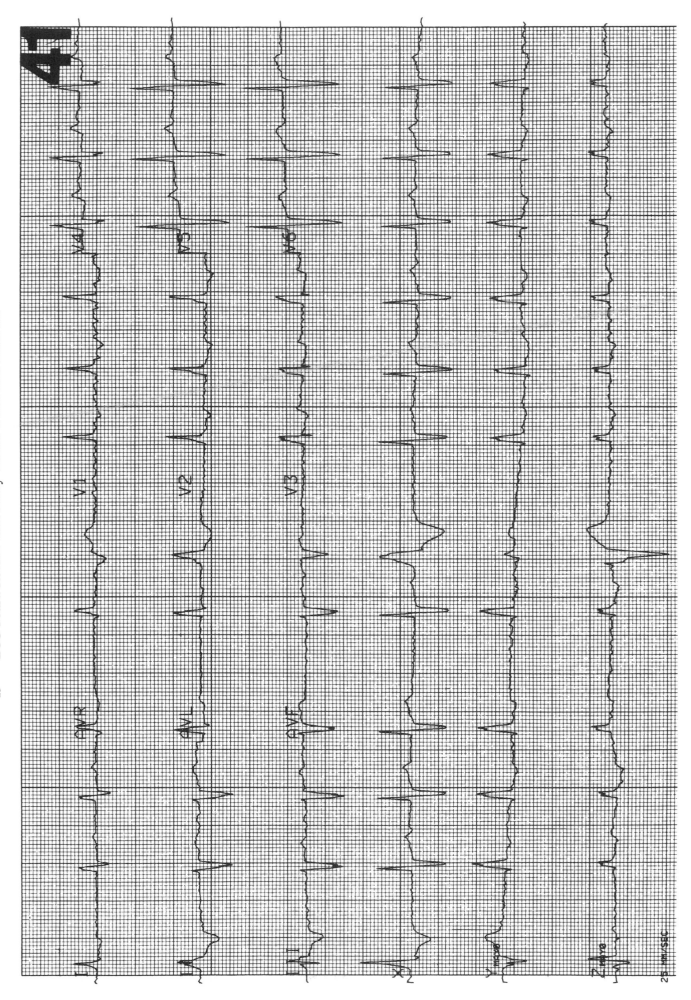

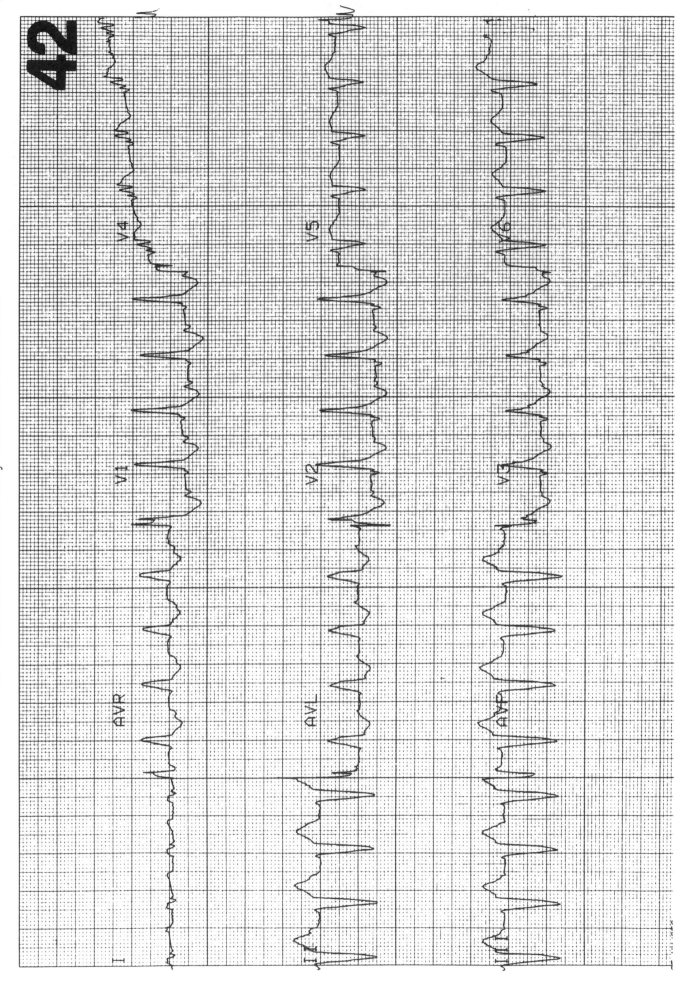

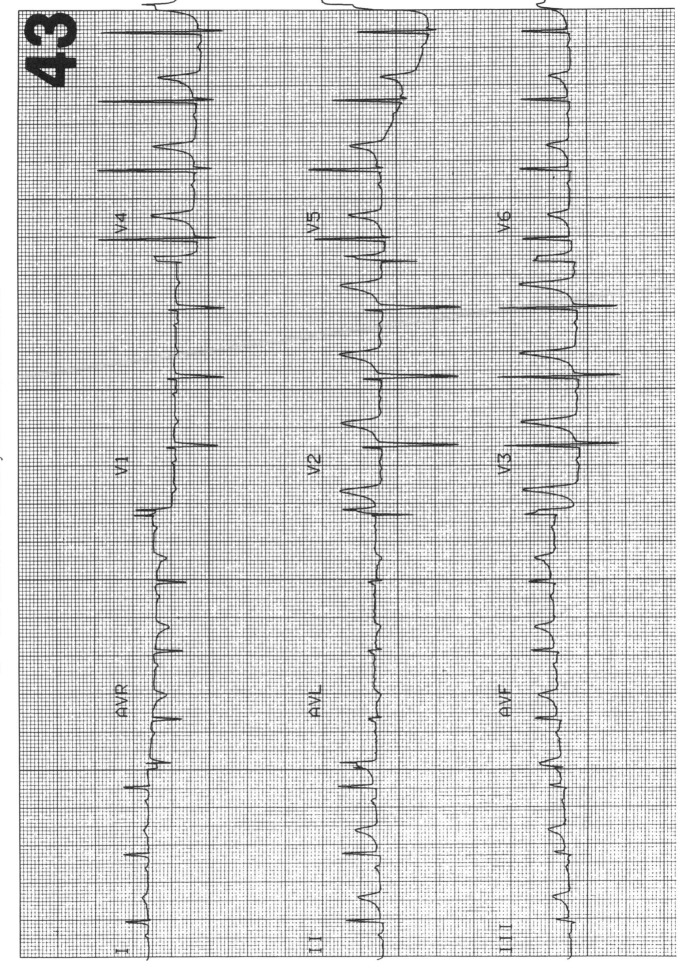

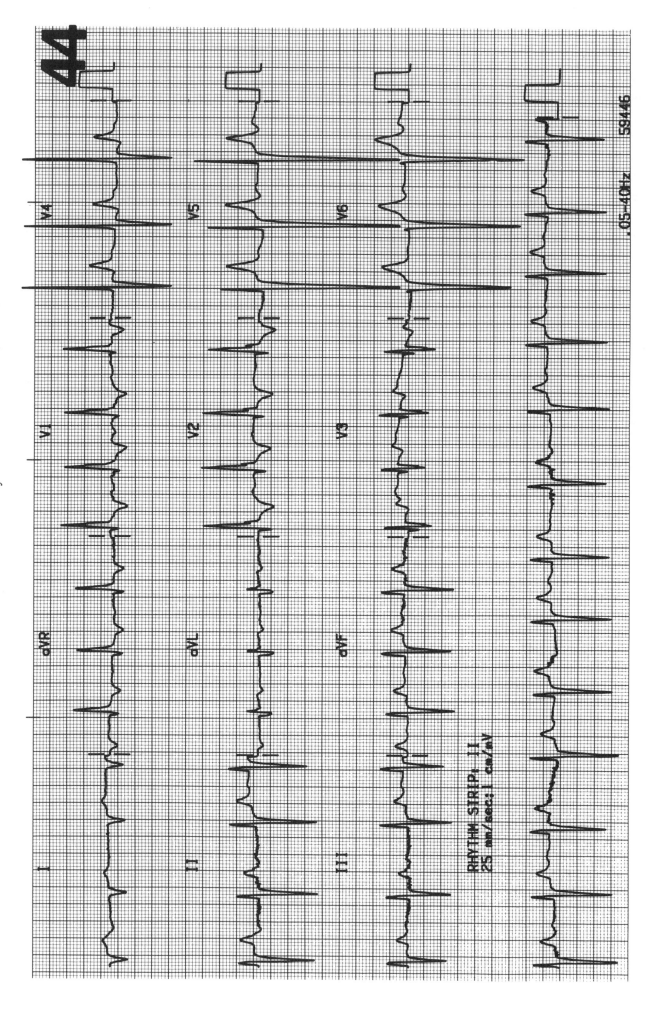

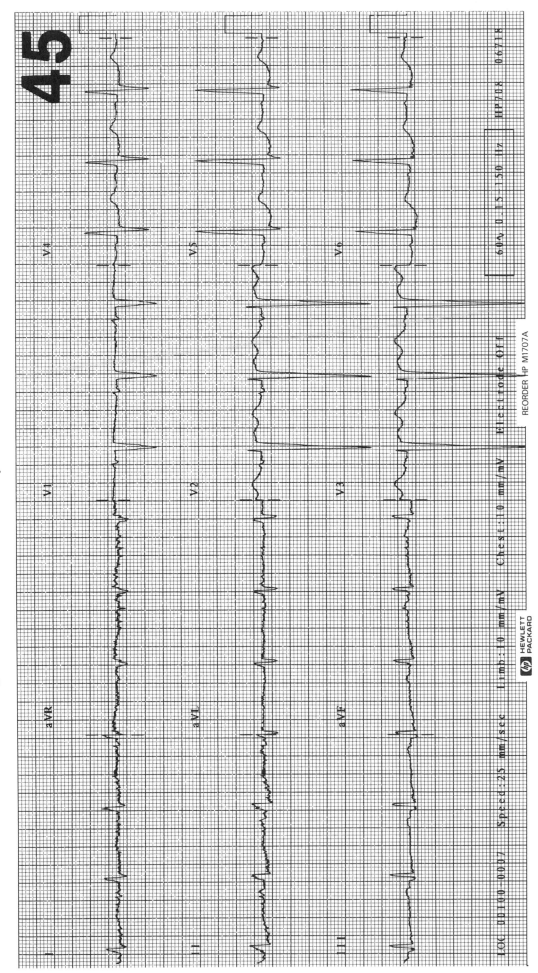

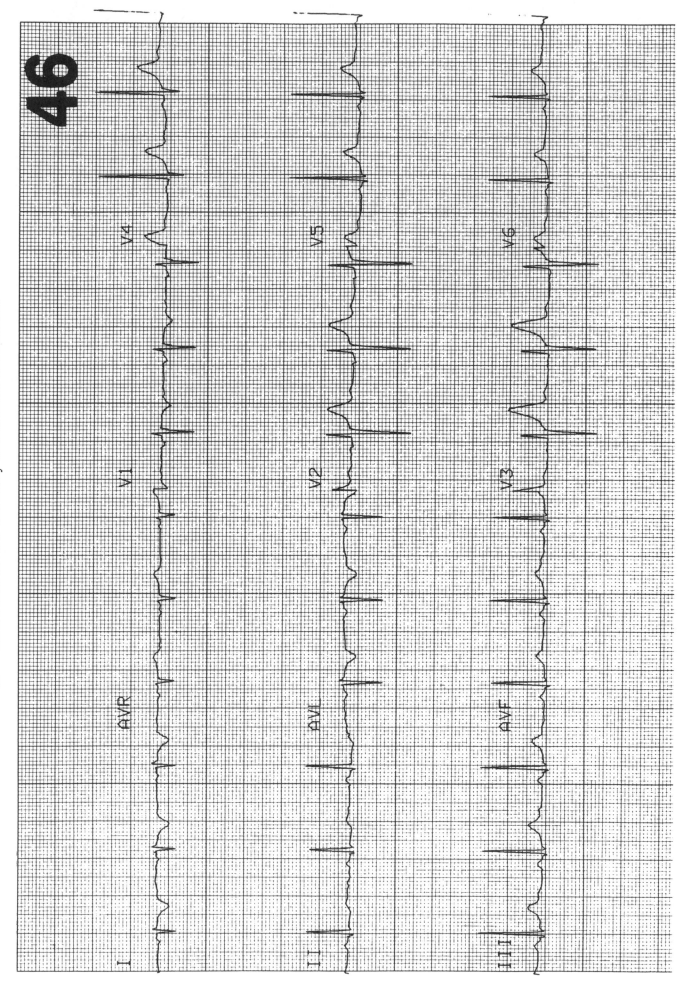

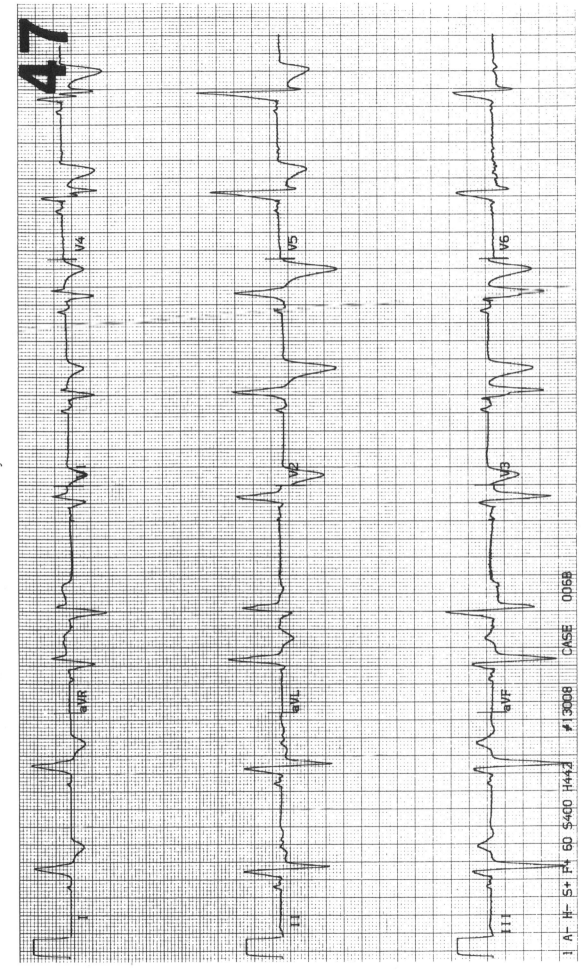

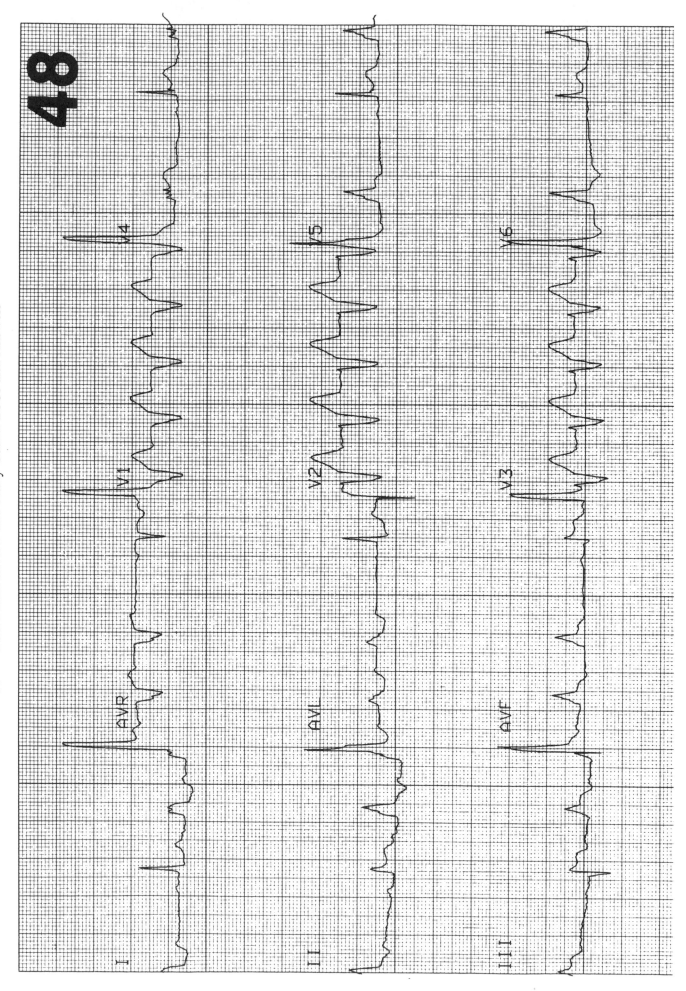

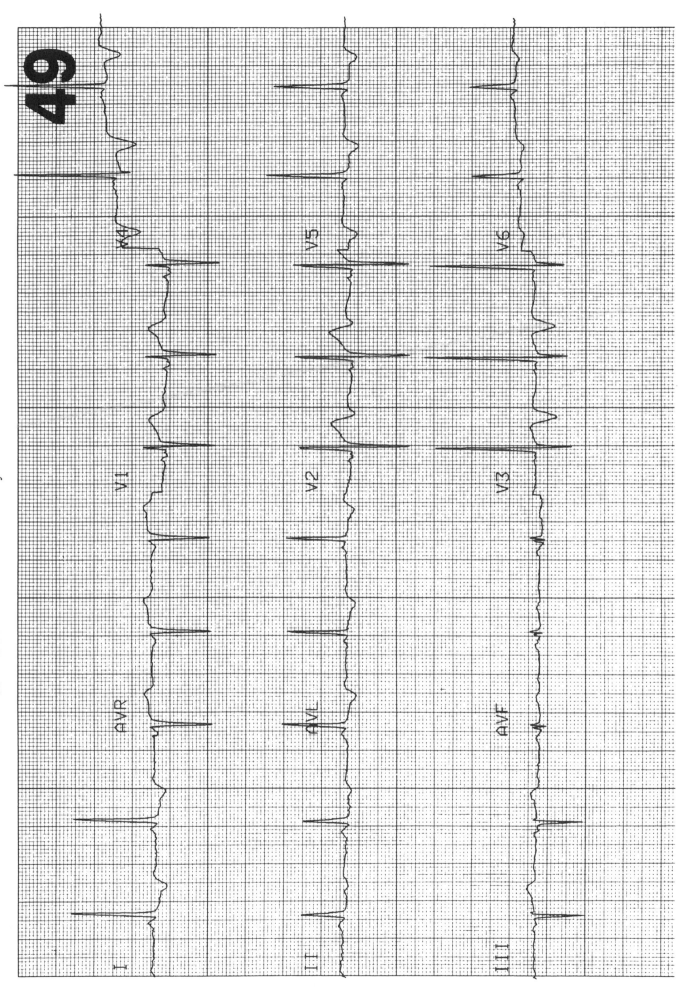

50

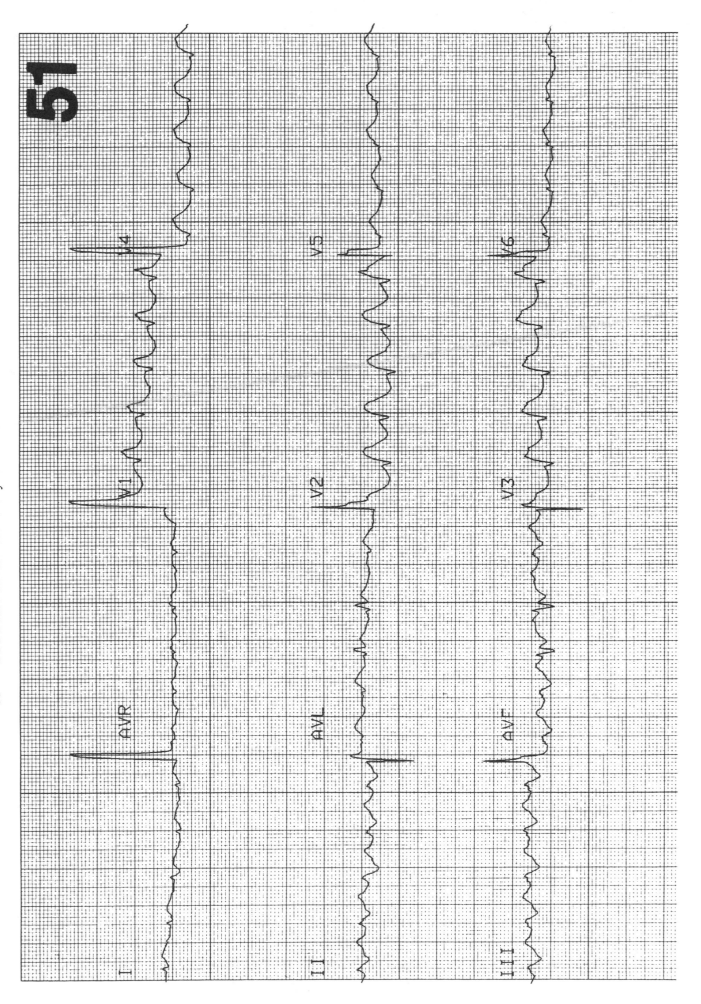

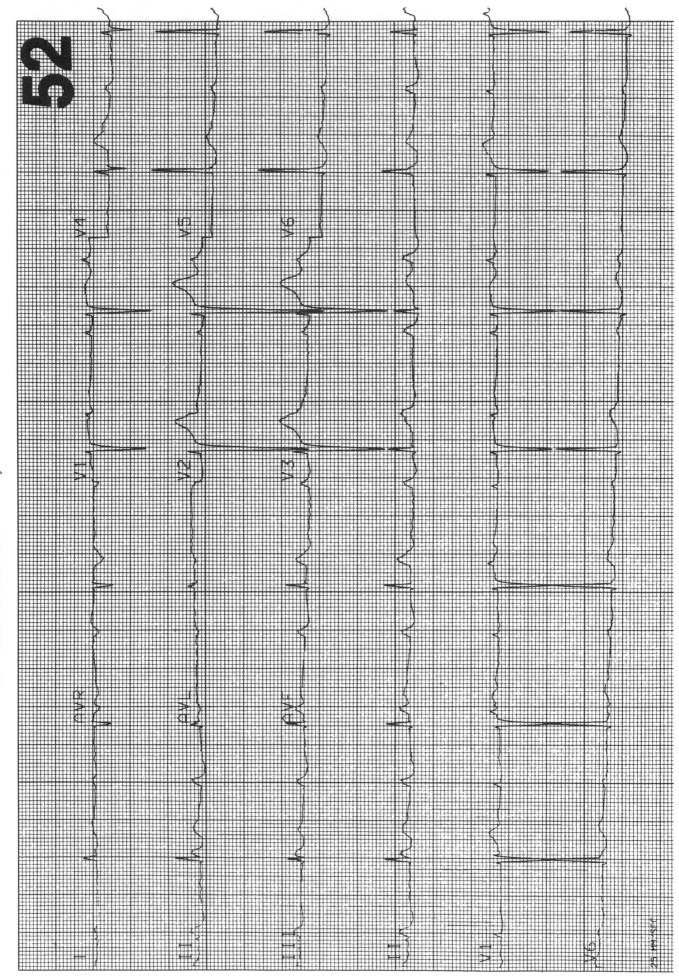

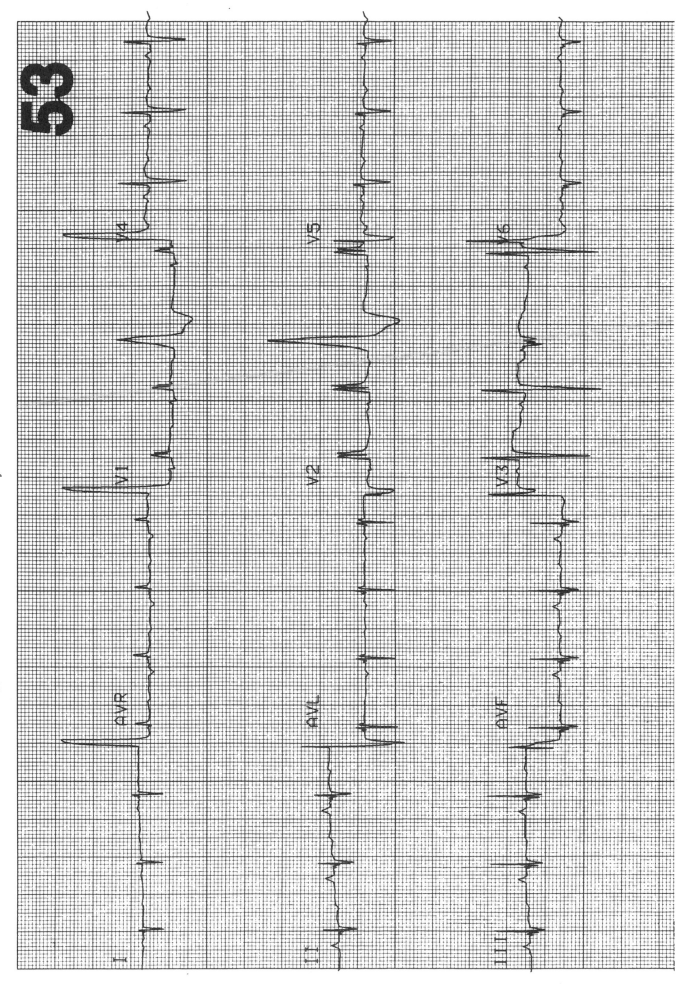

54

55

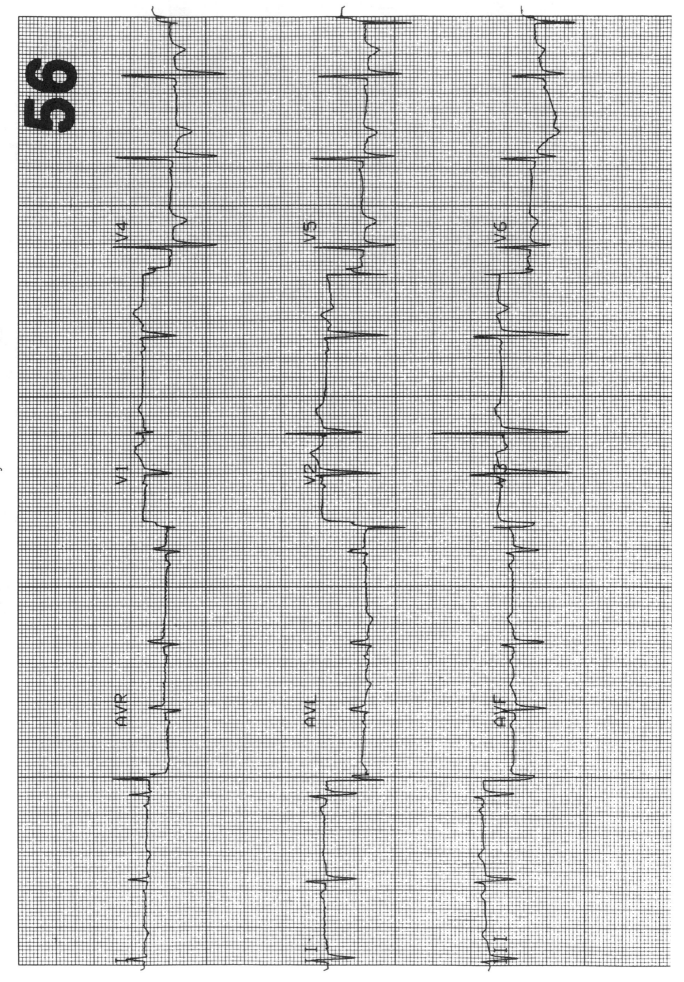

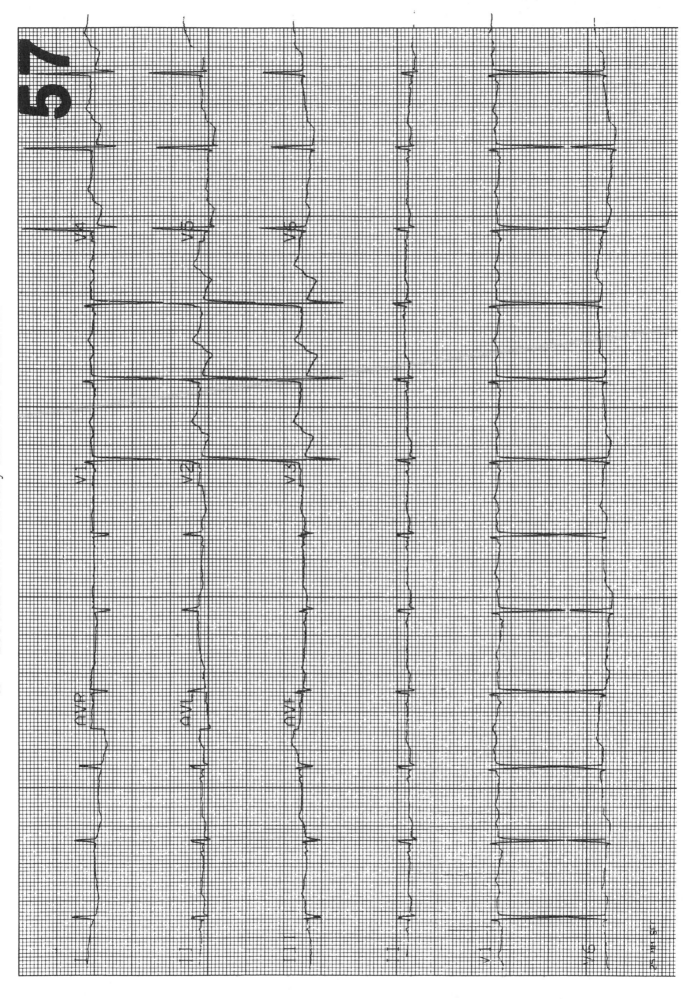

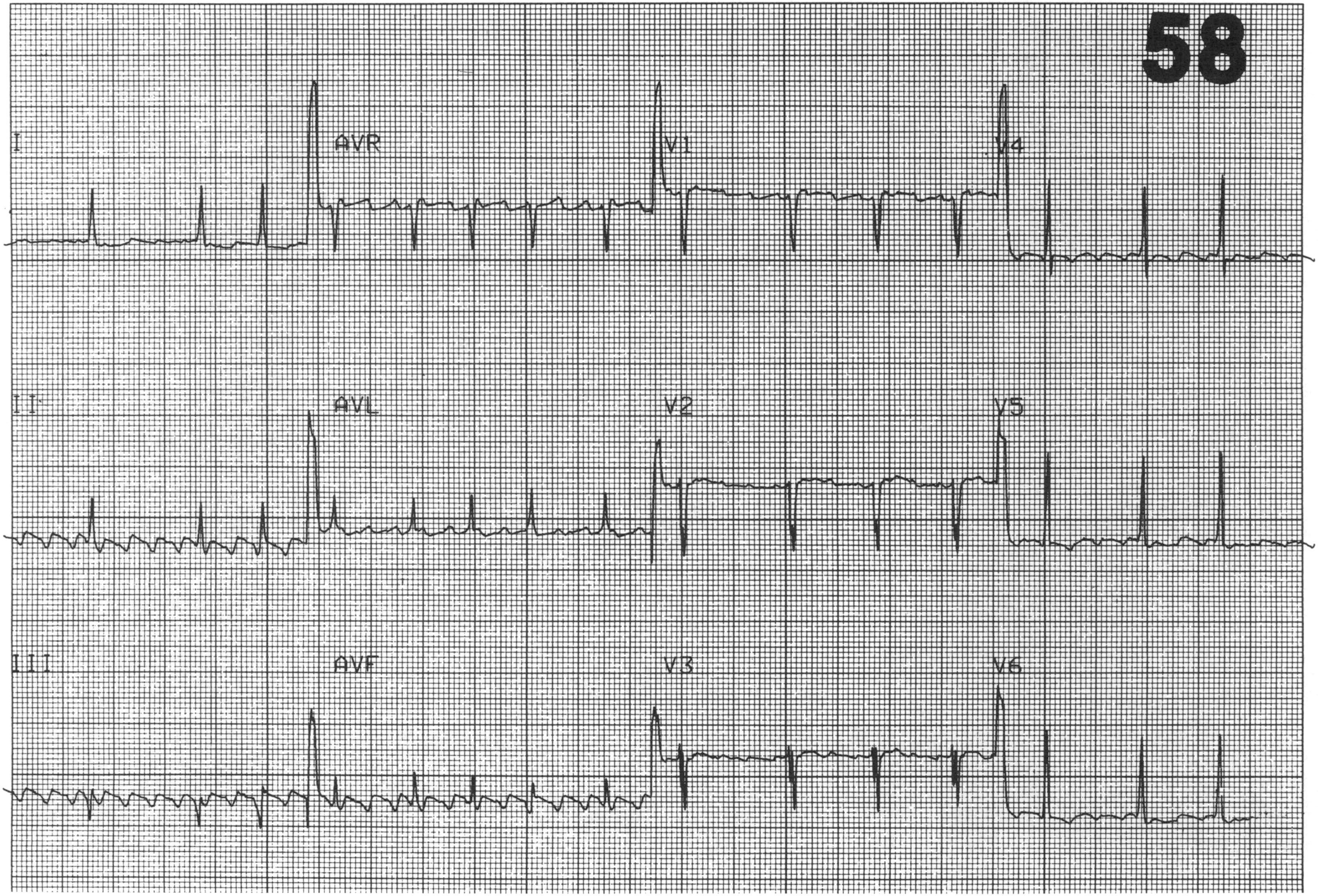
58
I
AVR
V1
V4
II
AVL
V2
V5
III
AVF
V3
V6

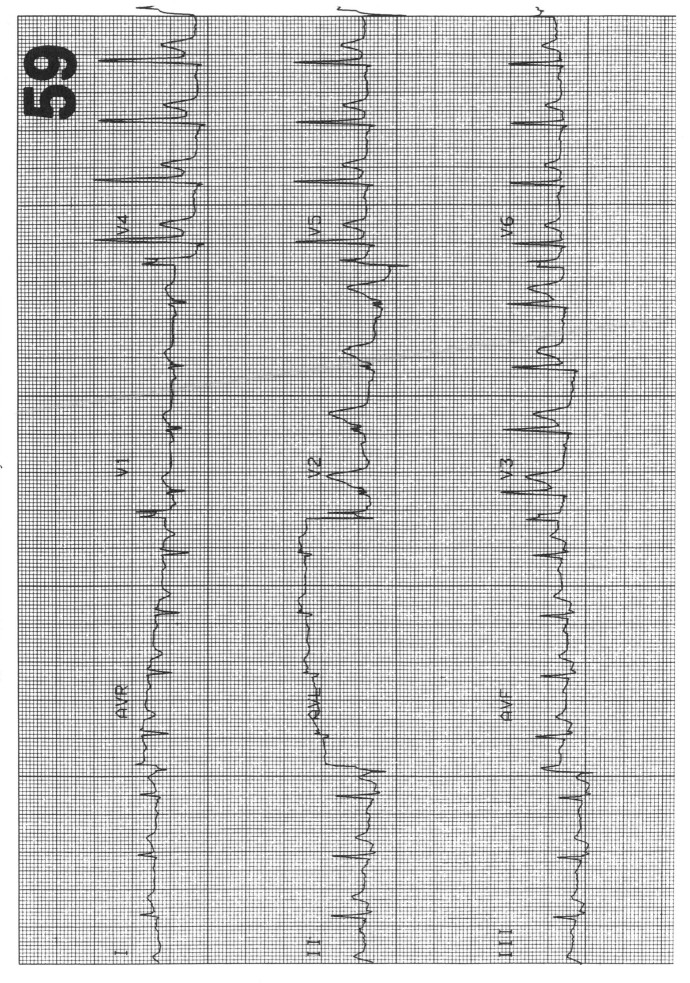

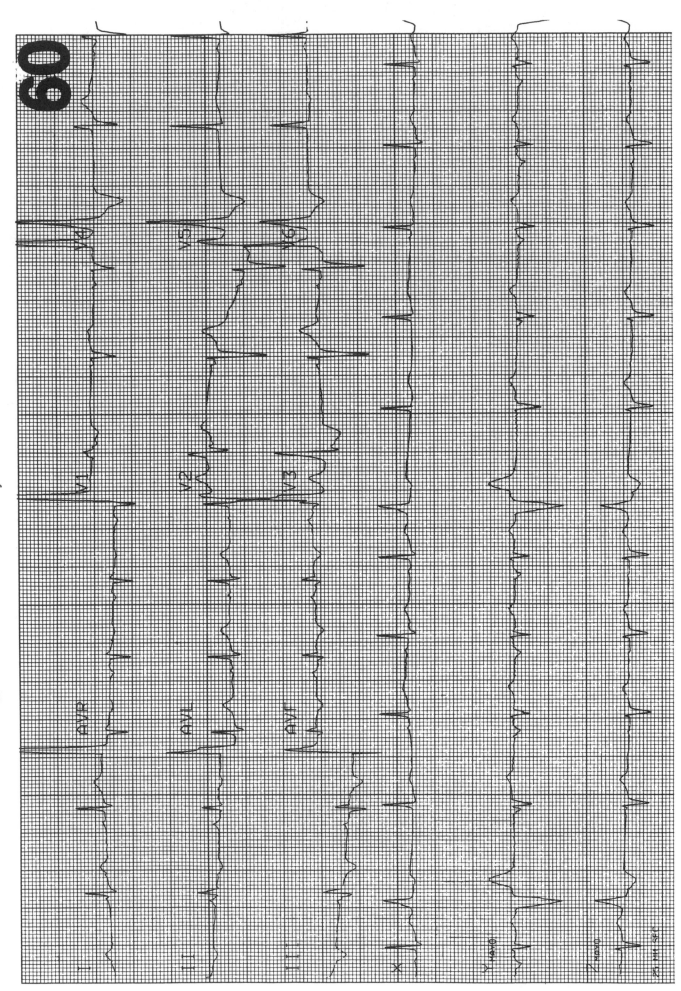

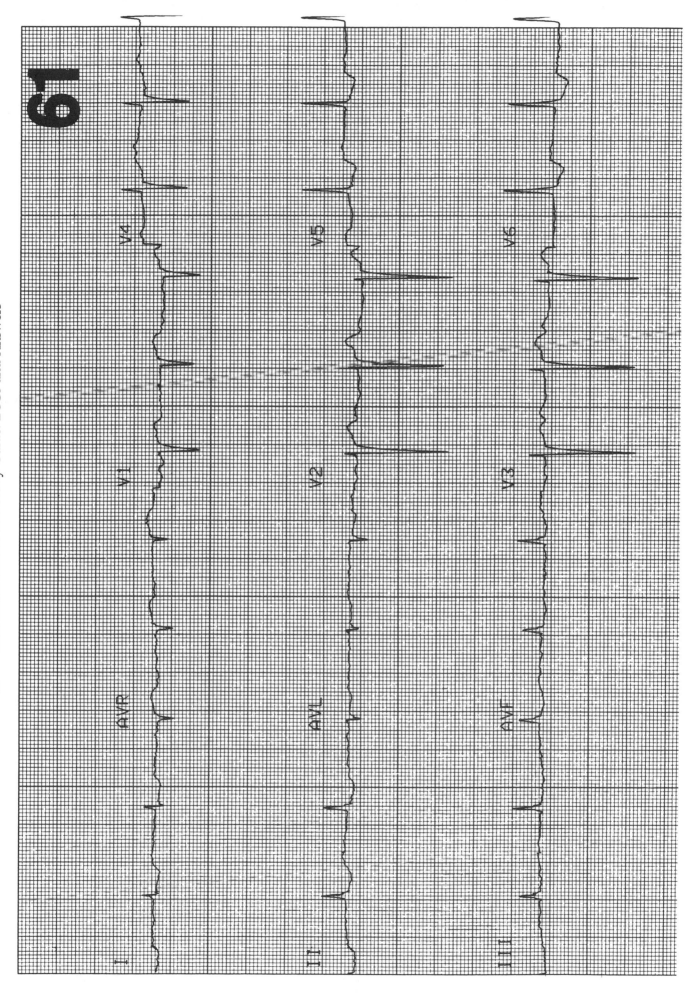

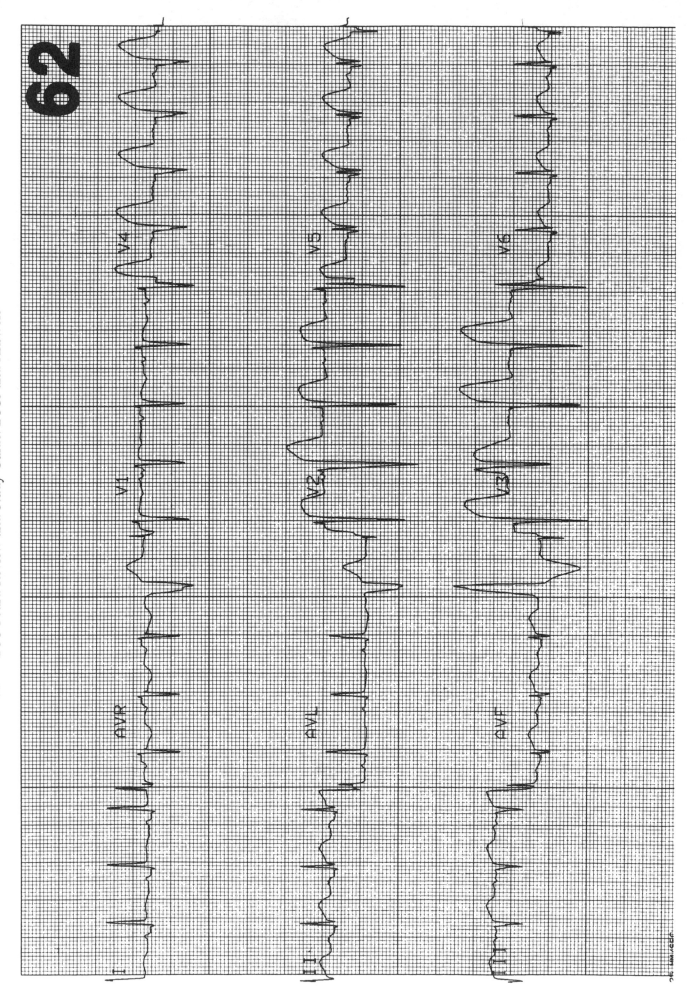

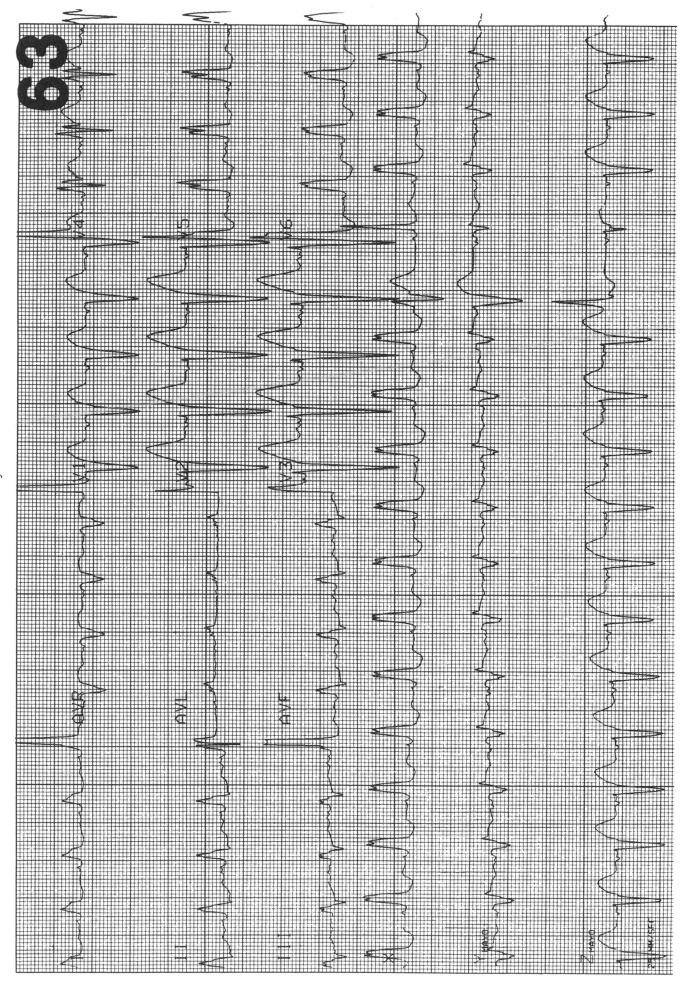

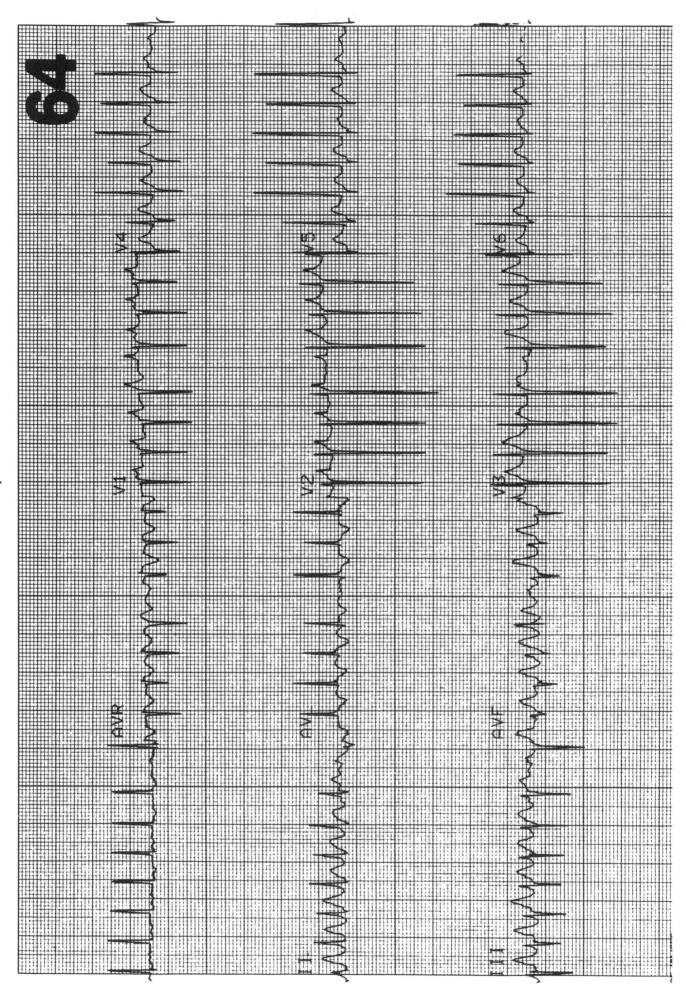

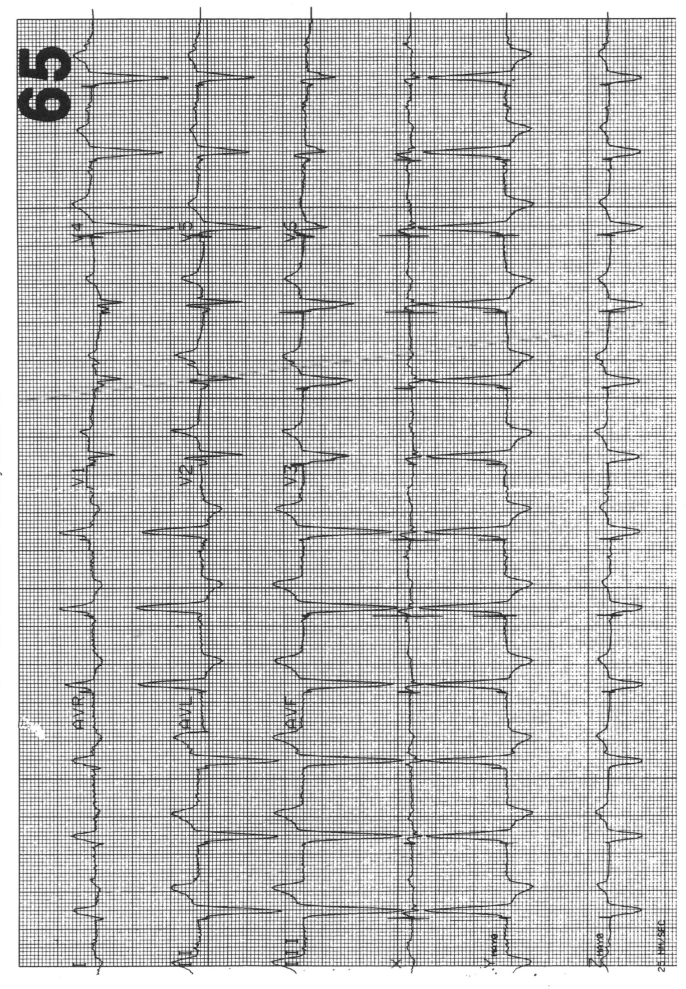

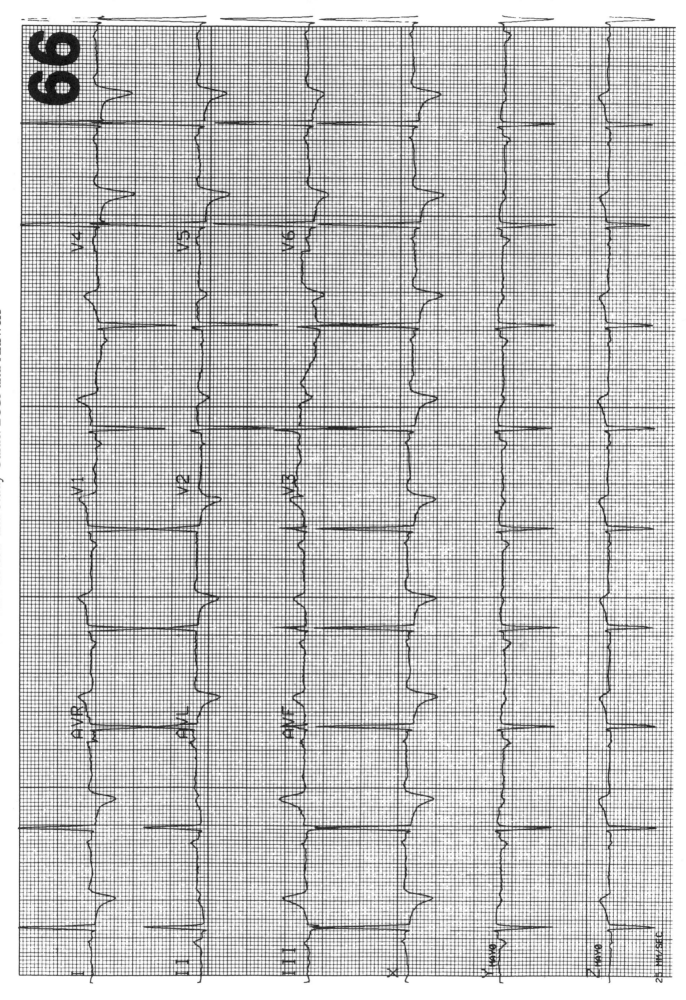

67

aVR*   V1 *
*

aVL*   V2 *
*

aVF*   V3 *
*

II

Raw Rhythm   Computer Synthesized Rhythm

81 A+ H- S+ F+ 60 S400 H442 #13 81   CASE   006B   * — Computer Synthesized Rhythm

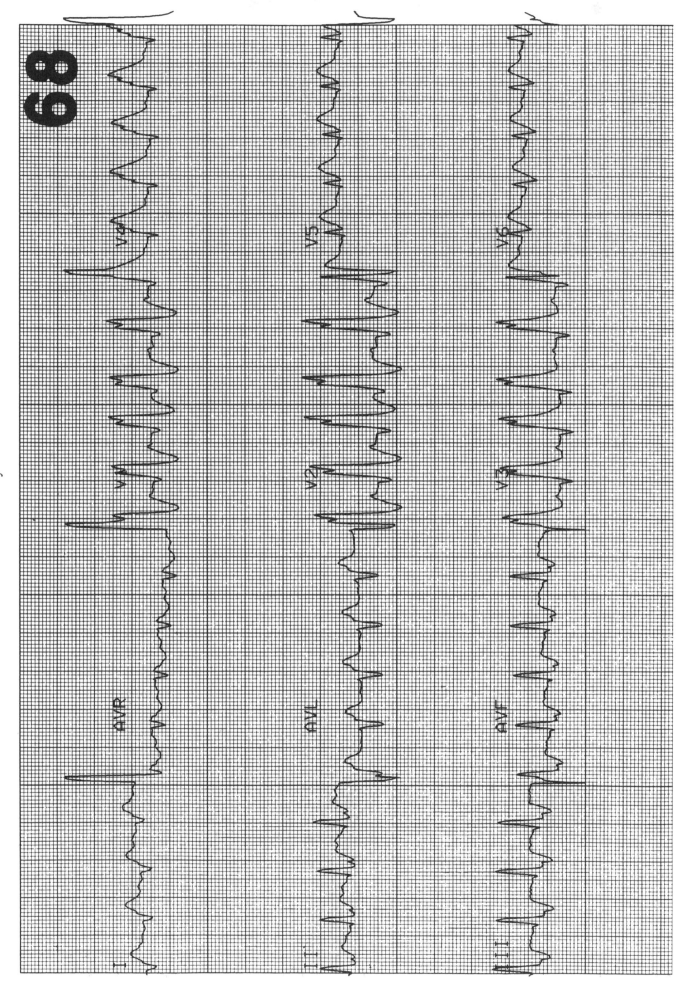

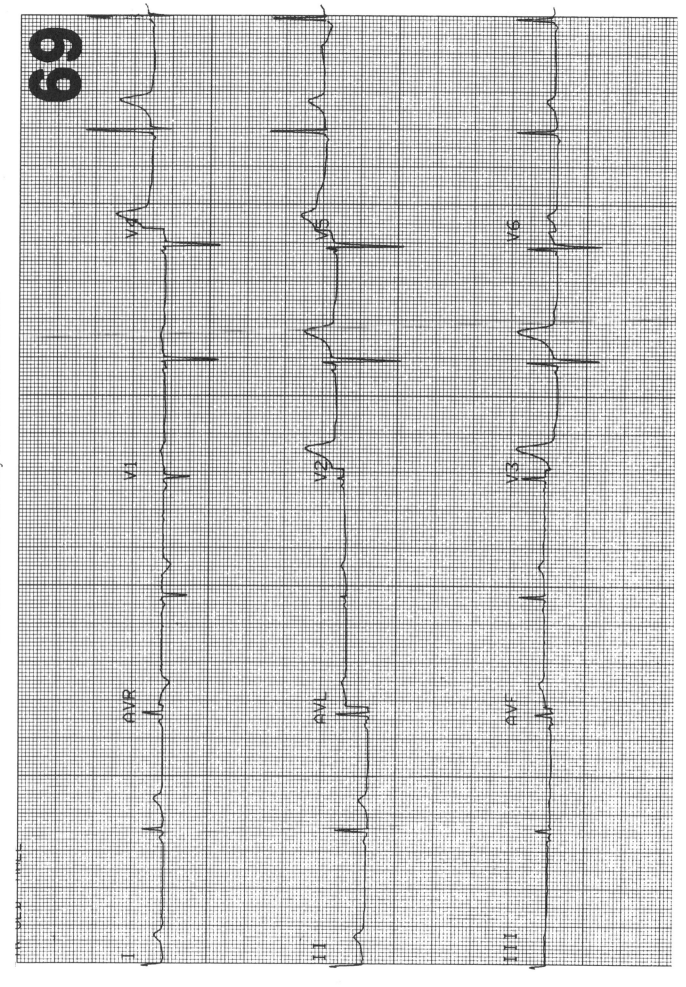

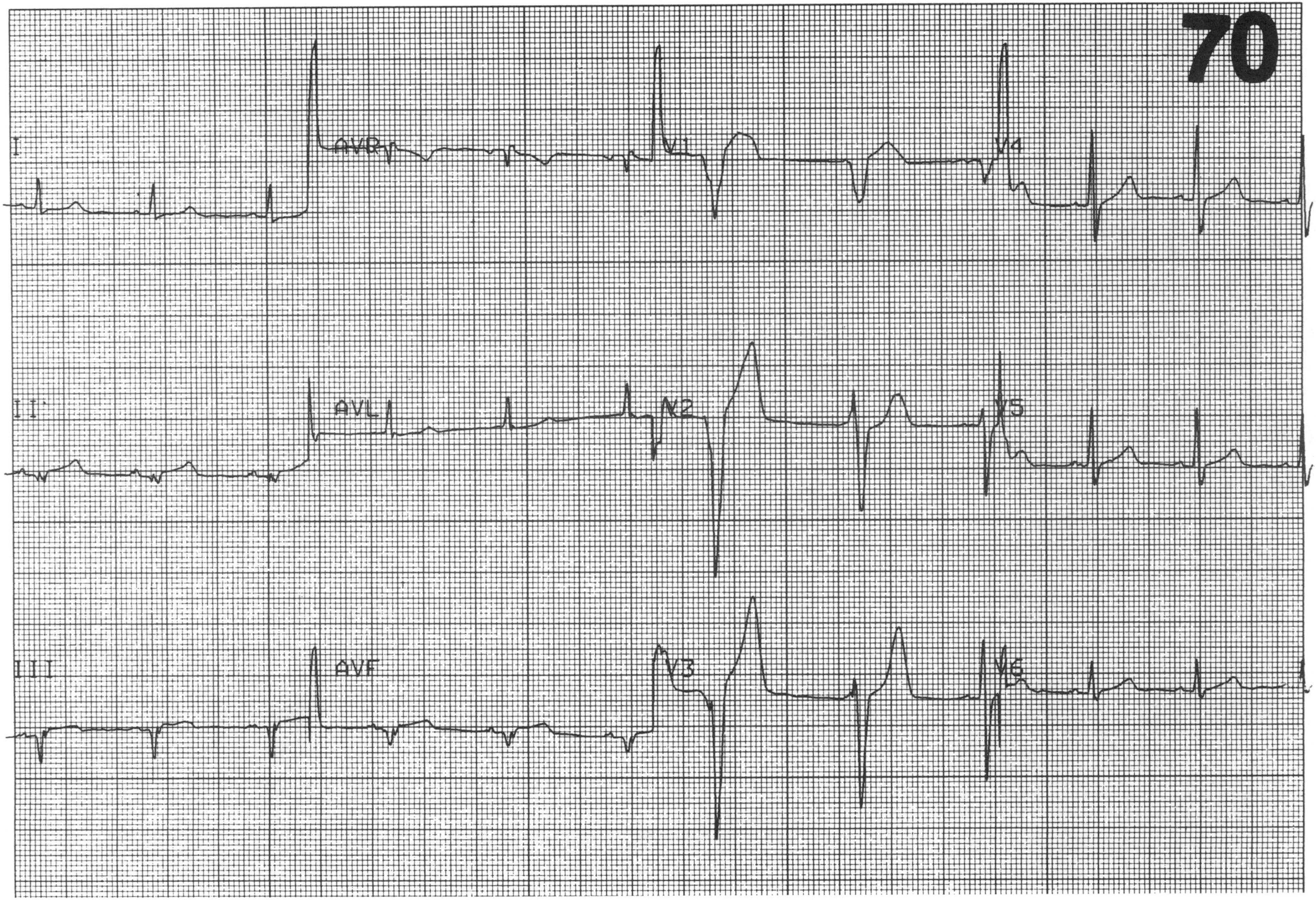
70
I
AVR
V1
V4
II
AVL
V2
V5
III
AVF
V3
V6

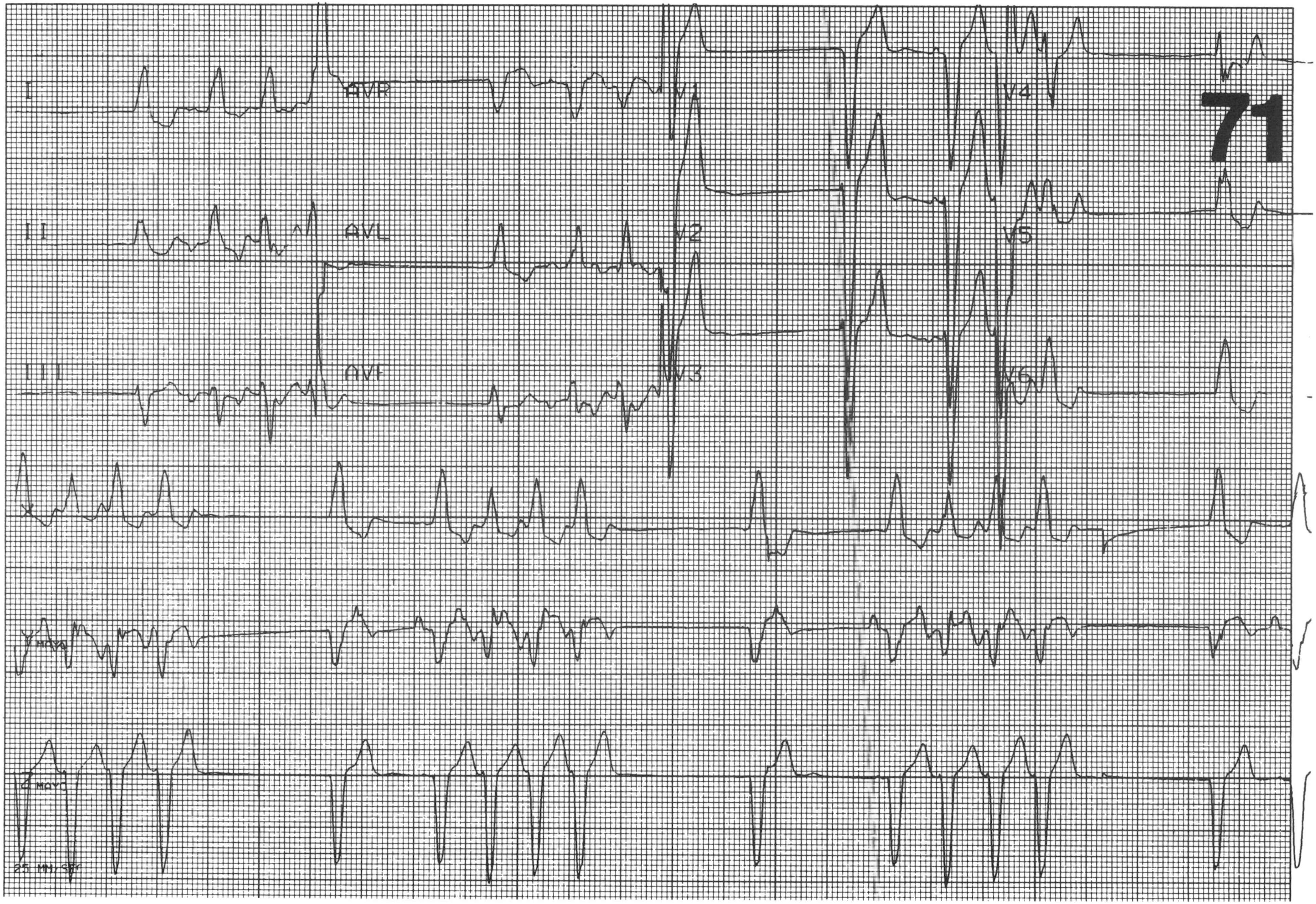

71
I
II
III
AVR
AVL
AVF
V1
V2
V3
V4
V5
V6
25 MM/SEC

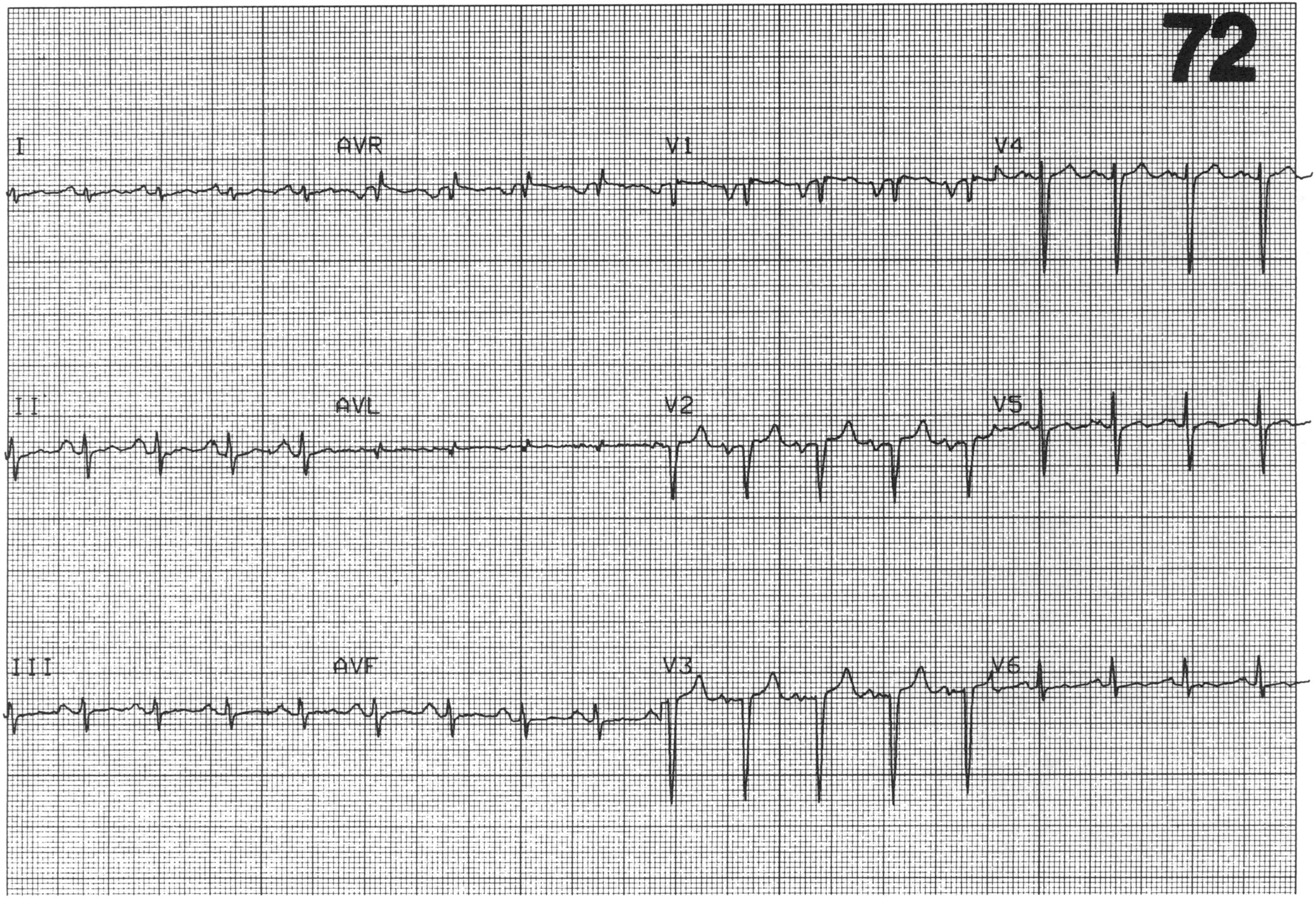
72
I
AVR
V1
V4
II
AVL
V2
V5
III
AVF
V3
V6

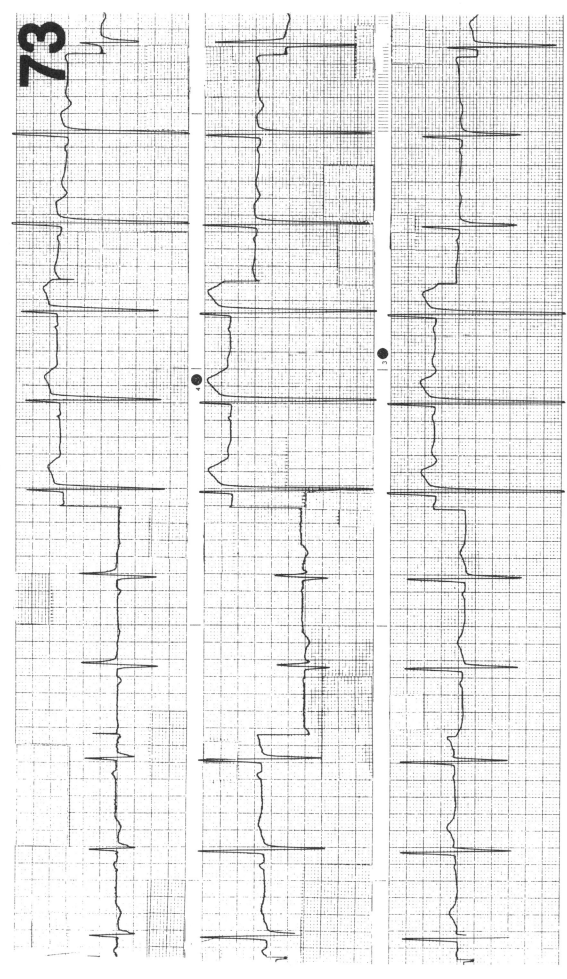

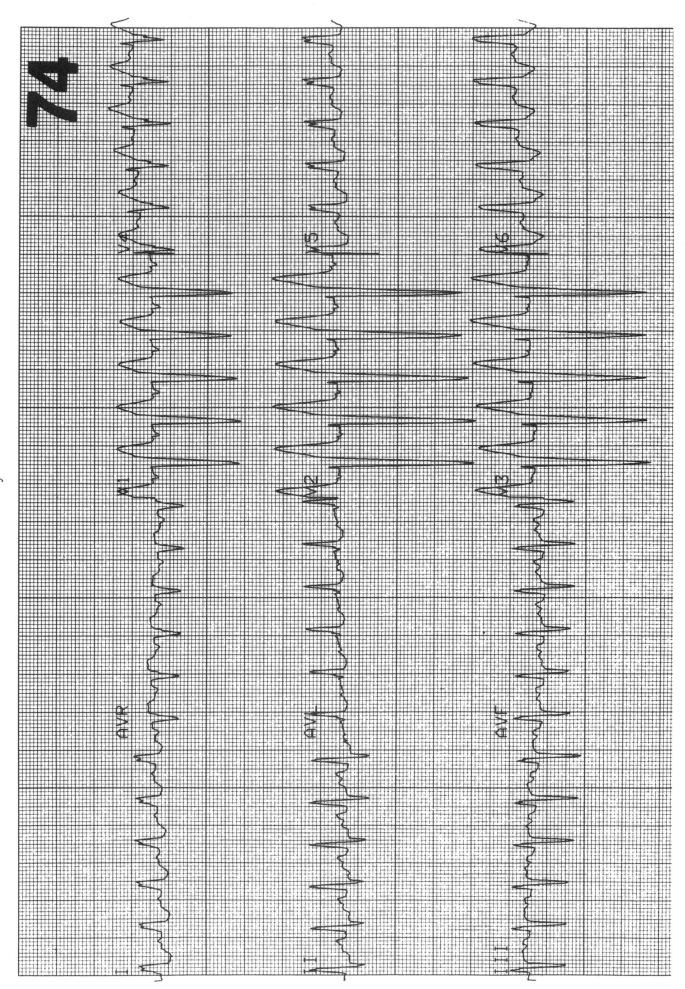

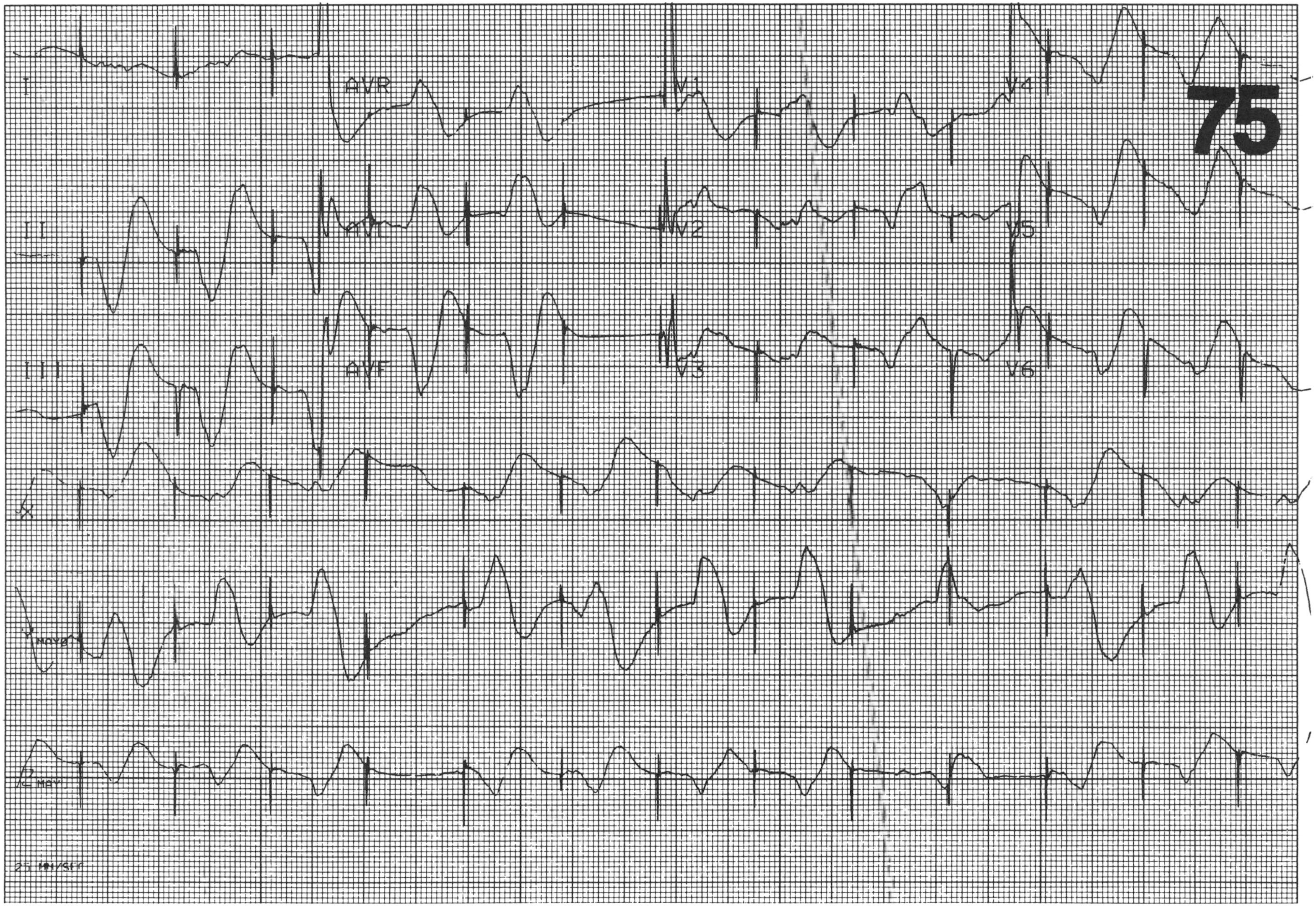
75
I
AVR
V1
V4
II
AVL
V2
V5
III
AVF
V3
V6
25 MM/SEC

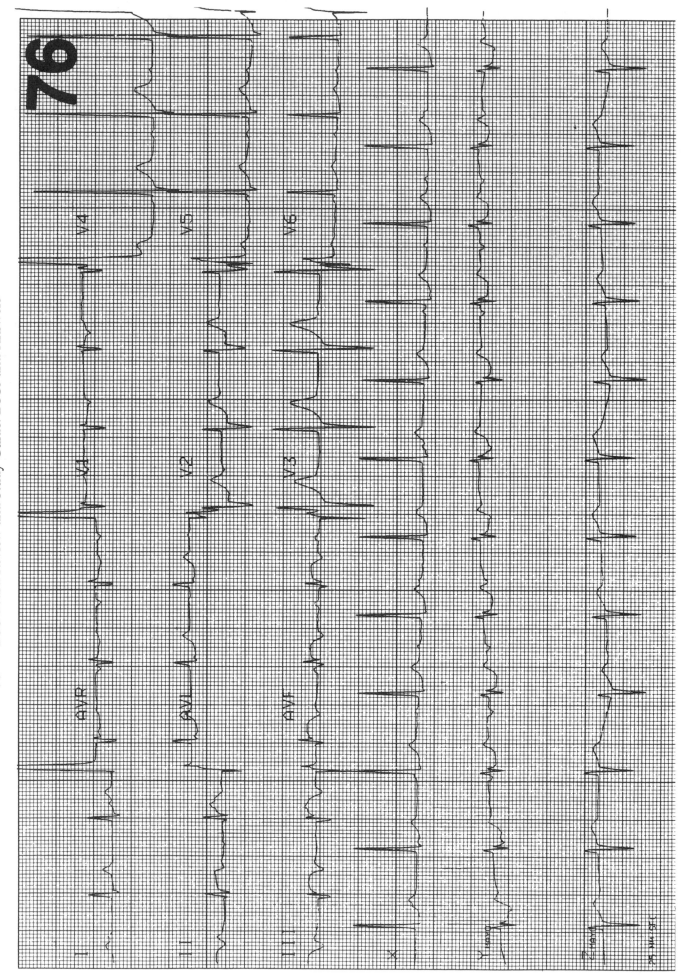

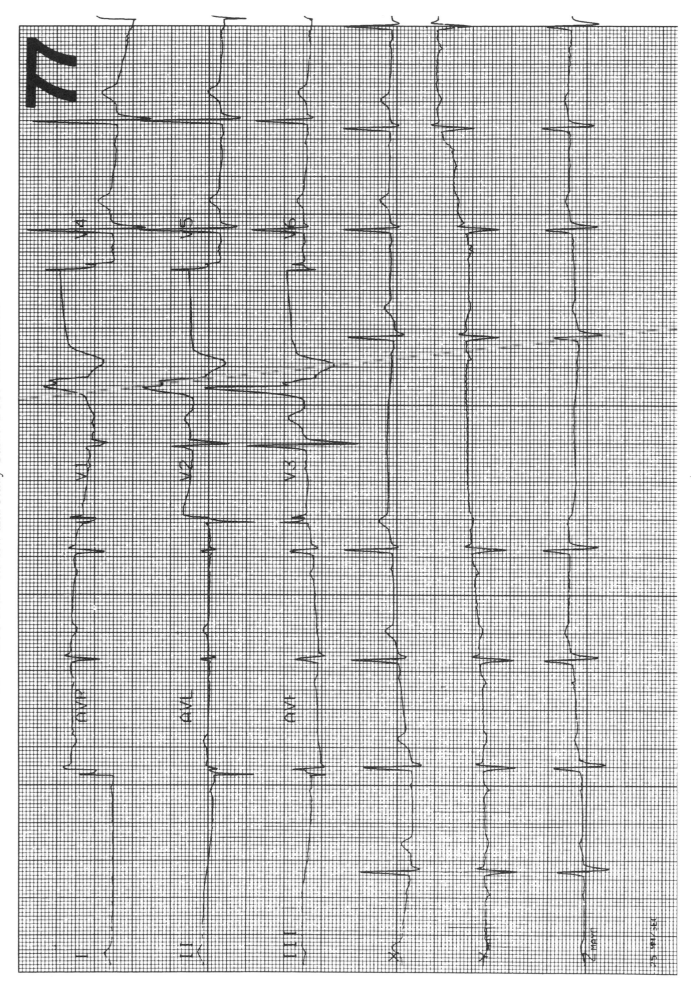

78

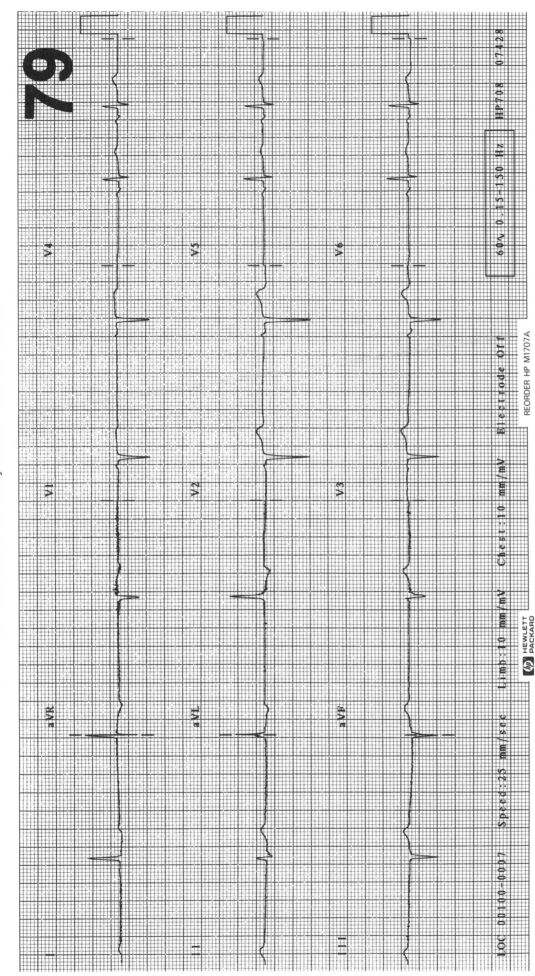

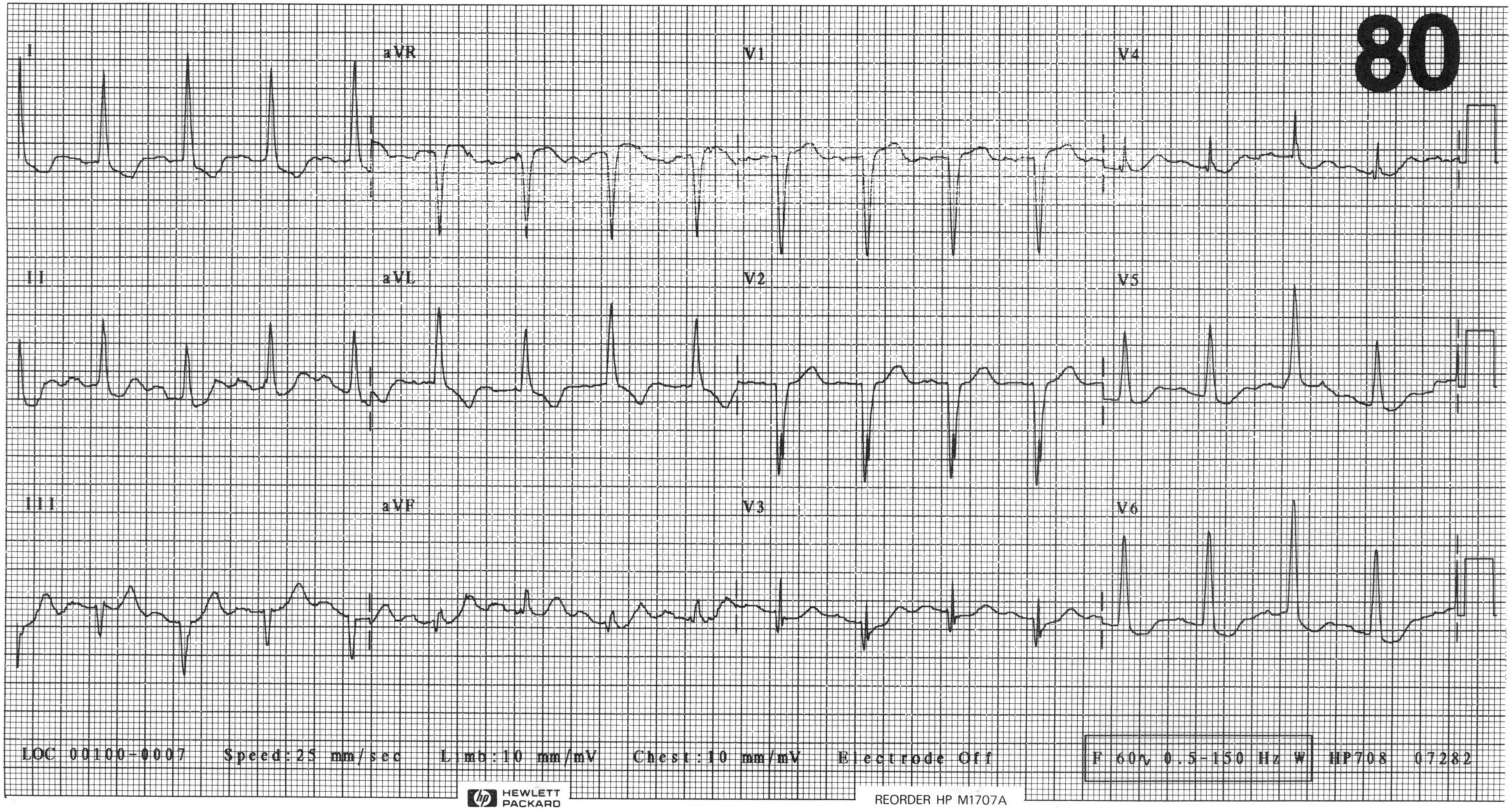
80
I
aVR
V1
V4
II
aVL
V2
V5
III
aVF
V3
V6
LOC 00100-0007 Speed:25 mm/sec Limb:10 mm/mV Chest:10 mm/mV Electrode Off
F 60∿ 0.5-150 Hz W HP708 07282
HEWLETT PACKARD
REORDER HP M1707A

Answers

1. This ECG shows sinus tachycardia with low voltage in both the limb and precordial chest leads. There are Q waves in leads V_1 through V_3 compatible with an anteroseptal myocardial infarction. There are mild nondiagnostic ST-T abnormalities particularly in the anterolateral leads. The most notable feature is electrical alternans seen in several leads but particularly in leads V_1, V_4, and V_5. This combination of findings is quite suggestive of pericardial effusion.

(Answers: 2d, 9b, 9e, 11i, 12c, 14o)

2. This tracing shows an atrial rhythm at approximately 97 bpm with an accelerated AV junctional rhythm noted. The rhythm is most likely junctional because of the narrow QRS complexes. AV dissociation is noted in several leads. However, the junctional rhythm is not totally regular, suggesting that there are capture complexes at times. Nonspecific ST-T wave abnormalities are present diffusely. Although there are high voltage QRS complexes, definitive criteria for left ventricular hypertrophy are not clearly met.

(Answers: 2g, 3c, 5c, 5d, 12c)

3. This tracing shows sinus rhythm at slightly greater than 100 bpm. There is third degree AV block with an accelerated AV junctional rhythm. Q waves and ST segment elevation in the inferior leads are diagnostic for a recent or probably acute inferior wall infarction due to coronary artery disease. Prominent negative component of P waves in lead V_1 is suggestive of left atrial abnormality.

(Answers: 2d, 3c, 6e, 8b, 11e, 12e, 14r)

4. This tracing shows a wide complex tachycardia with left axis deviation. The most notable diagnostic feature is a capture complex seen in the third QRS complex in leads V_4–V_6. Ventricular concordance is also present. These findings are suggestive of ventricular tachycardia.

(Answers: 4f, 5c, 9c)

5. This ECG shows a normal sinus rhythm. There is a short PR interval and prominent delta waves with a prolonged QRS duration and with an inferior

pseudo-infarction pattern. This is compatible with Wolff-Parkinson-White syndrome. Fusion between normal and pre-excited complexes is present. Mild anterior ST-T abnormalities are noted, probably secondary to the pre-excitation.

(Answers: 2a, 5a, 6h, 12g)

6. This subtle ECG shows probable ectopic atrial rhythm with a nonspecific atrial abnormality and an abnormal P wave axis. Upright P waves in leads III and F suggest that it is sinus or rising high in the atrium. There is an accelerated AV junctional rhythm with isorhythmic AV dissociation noted particularly in the rhythm strips. The axis is deviated to the right and criteria for right ventricular hypertrophy are met. Specifically, there is right axis deviation, a prominent R wave in lead V_1, and an S greater than R wave in lead V_6. Anterior ST-T abnormalities are probably due to hypertrophy.

(Answers: 2g, 3c, 5d, 8c, 9d, 10c, 12g)

7. This tracing shows a normal sinus rhythm. The axis and intervals are normal and there is a normal QRS and T wave contour compatible with normal electrocardiogram. During lead switches, the artifact is so fed that should not be confused with ectopic beats.

(Answer: 1a)

8. This tracing shows a normal sinus rhythm. There is an abnormal P wave noted in lead V_1 compatible with nonspecific atrial abnormality. The most notable feature is prominent R waves in leads V_1 and V_2 compatible with posterior infarction. There is ST segment elevation in the inferior leads that would make other possibilities for prominent anterior R waves less likely. Coronary artery disease is very likely to be present.

(Answers: 2a, 8c, 11e, 11f, 12e, 14r)

9. The most notable feature of this ECG is the rhythm. This is best seen on the rhythm strips, particularly in lead X. There is a sinus rhythm with an accelerated idioventricular rhythm and variable AV block. Capture complexes are noted at times as well as a fusion complex. AV block is present but variable.

(Answers: 2a, 4g, 5a, 5c, 6f)

10. This important ECG is diagnostic for Wolff-Parkinson-White syndrome. There is a rapid irregular wide complex tachycardia with ventricular rates up to 300 bpm due to atrial fibrillation. There are variable degrees of pre-excitation and ST-T abnormalities due to the intraventricular conduction disturbance from pre-excitation.

(Answers: 2s, 5a, 6h, 7i, 12g)

11. This typical ECG shows sinus rhythm with Wolff-Parkinson-White syndrome and prominent delta waves. Fusion complexes between normally conducted and pre-excited beats are noted. ST-T abnormalities are noted due to intraventricular conduction disturbance.

(Answers: 2a, 5a, 6h, 12g)

12. The rhythm is the most notable feature of this ECG. There are inverted P waves in the inferior leads compatible with retrograde atrial activation. The PR interval is short, suggesting junctional origin of the rhythm. The rate is 80 bpm, which would suggest an accelerated junctional rhythm. Peaked T waves are present, and are consistent with hyperkalemia.

(Answers: 2t, 3c, 12j, 14e)

13. This ECG shows a baseline artifact in a repetitive pattern that may be due to tremor. Peaked inferior P waves are suggestive of right atrial abnormality. The prominent negative component P wave in lead V_1 also is quite suggestive of left atrial abnormality. There is first degree AV block with left ventricular hypertrophy by voltage criteria. A typical strain pattern is not present. There is ST elevation in the anterolateral or apical leads suggestive of an injury pattern.

(Answers: 1d, 2d, 6a, 8a, 8b, 10a, 11a, 12e, 14r)

14. Mitral stenosis is strongly suggested by this ECG. The combination of right axis deviation, right atrial abnormality, and a prominent R wave in lead V_1 is suggestive of right ventricular hypertrophy. Left atrial abnormality is also quite prominent with a wide P wave in the inferior leads with notching. In addition, there is a prominent negative component to the P wave in lead V_1. The combination of left atrial enlargement and right ventricular hypertrophy is suggestive but not diagnostic of mitral stenosis. First degree AV block is also present.

(Answers: 2d, 6a, 8a, 8b, 9d, 10c, 12g, 14l)

15. Combined ventricular hypertrophy is present in this ECG. There are high voltage QRS complexes with right axis deviation. In addition, the Kutzner-Wachtel phenomenon is present, with high voltage equiphasic complexes in the mid-precordial leads. Left atrial abnormality B is also noted. Finally, there are ST-T segment abnormalities secondary to hypertrophy as well as prominent U waves that are nonspecific.

(Answers: 2a, 8b, 9d, 10d, 12g, 12l)

16. This ECG shows atrial fibrillation with frequent examples of aberrant intraventricular conduction (Ashman's phenomenon). The wide QRS complexes are in an irregular pattern and have a right bundle branch block configuration, making ventricular tachycardia quite unlikely. There are nonspecific ST-T wave abnormalities. The narrow QRS complexes do show an age-indeterminate inferior infarction suggestive of coronary artery disease.

(Answers: 2s, 7i, 11k, 12c, 12g, 14r)

17. The most notable feature of this ECG is the negative P wave and QRS complex in lead I. There are two diagnostic possibilities for this abnormality: dextrocardia or limb lead reversal. The diminishing R wave across the precordium from V_1 through V_6 confirms the diagnosis of dextrocardia.

(Answers: 2a, 9d, 12c, 14k)

18. Tall peaked inferior P waves are diagnostic for right atrial enlargement. There is also a prominent negative P component in V_1 suggestive of left atrial enlargement. There is right axis deviation with probable right ventricular

hypertrophy. S wave is significantly larger than R wave in lead V_6. Finally, there is poor anterior R wave progression. These findings are typical of severe chronic obstructive lung disease with hyperinflation and pulmonary hypertension.

(Answers: 2d, 8a, 8b, 9d, 10c, 12g, 14m)

19. Pacemaker spikes are present and are capturing the atrium. Normal conduction through the AV node results in intrinsic QRS complexes (QRS width = 120 ms). There is not a typical right or left bundle branch block configuration, thus yielding a diagnosis of nonspecific intraventricular conduction disturbance. A single ventricular premature complex is noted in leads I, II, and III. Finally, ST segment elevation in leads V_2–V_5 is suggestive of but not diagnostic for myocardial injury (specificity is reduced in the presence of intraventricular conduction defect).

(Answers: 4a, 6a, 7h, 12g, 13a)

20. This ECG shows sinus rhythm with complete left bundle branch block. QRS duration is greater than 120 ms and there is a delayed intrinsicoid deflection in the left precordial leads and in lead I. Q waves are present in leads I and aVL, but are nondiagnostic in the setting of left bundle branch block.

(Answers: 2a, 7f, 12g, 14r)

21. This ECG shows sinus rhythm with third degree AV block. A wide complex escape rhythm with a rate less than 30 bpm is present and is quite typical for a ventricular escape rhythm. P wave duration is 120 ms with a prominent negative component in lead V_1 diagnostic of a left atrial abnormality.

(Answers: 2a, 4h, 6e, 8b)

22. The rhythm is the most notable feature of this ECG. An aberrantly conducted atrial premature complex is followed by AV dissociation and a wide QRS complex escape rhythm typical for a ventricular rhythm. The penultimate beat of the tracing is a fusion beat followed by resumption of a typical QRS complex. The native QRS complex shows left axis deviation with a right bundle branch block configuration. There is probable left

anterior fascicular block. Left atrial abnormality is present with a wide P wave with a prominent negative component in lead V_1. There are nondiagnostic ST-T abnormalities, probably due to intraventricular conduction disturbance. In the limb leads, first degree AV block is apparent.

(Answers: 2c, 2i, 4h, 5a, 5d, 6a, 7b, 7c, 8b, 9c, 12g)

23. This tracing shows a normal sinus rhythm with normal axis and intervals. There is J point elevation in the anterior leads typical of early repolarization pattern (a normal variant).

(Answers: 1b, 2a, 12a)

24. The rhythm is irregular with atrial fibrillation most easily seen in leads II and aVF. The QRS complex is quite wide and bizarre, suggestive of severe metabolic abnormalities. These findings would be most consistent with hyperkalemia, however, other severe metabolic abnormalities or drug toxicities could result in this pattern also.

(Answers: 2s, 7h, 12g, 14e)

25. This ECG shows sinus tachycardia with polymorphic nonsustained ventricular tachycardia. Atrial activity and native QRS complexes are seen in leads aVR, aVL, aVF, and V_1–V_6. 2:1 AV block is noted in lead V_1. The atrial rate is approximately 140 bpm and is consistent with sinus tachycardia. Inferior ST segment elevation and small Q waves are noted, particularly in lead aVF with reciprocal anterolateral ST segment depression. Thus, an acute inferior and posterior infarction is probably responsible for the nonsustained ventricular tachycardia.

(Answers: 2d, 4f, 6d, 6f, 11e, 11f, 12e, 14r)

26. This ECG shows sinus tachycardia with no relationship between the QRS complexes and P waves, diagnostic of third degree AV block. Inferior P wave amplitude is 2.5 mV, yielding criteria for right atrial enlargement. There is a junctional escape rhythm. A prominent feature is inferior ST segment elevation compatible with injury pattern, which is likely responsible for the AV block. The ST segment depression in the anterior precordial leads is consistent with associated acute posterior injury. Coronary artery

disease should be scored as well. Because neither prominent R waves (anteriorly) are present yet, criteria are not met for acute infarction. An artifact is noted between the first and the second beats of the tracing, but does not appear to be related to tremor and thus does not warrant coding.

(Answers: 2d, 3d, 6e, 8a, 12e, 14r)

27. This tracing shows a sinus bradycardia with left axis deviation. A small Q wave in lead I and a large S wave in lead III are highly suggestive of a left anterior fascicular block. There is abnormal anterior R wave progression with loss of R waves moving from V_1 through V_3. This is highly suggestive for an anteroseptal infarction (although left anterior fascicular block can also result in low anterior forces). ST-T wave abnormalities are present suggestive of a recent event, and thus coronary artery disease is the likely cause. Left atrial abnormality is also noted in lead V_1.

(Answers: 2c, 7c, 8a, 9c, 11c, 12d, 14r)

28. This tracing shows a normal sinus rhythm with left axis deviation and possible left anterior fascicular block. The most notable features are Q waves in the high lateral and anterior leads and ST segment elevation compatible with extensive acute myocardial infarction.

(Answers: 2a, 7c, 9c, 11a, 11b, 11d, 12e, 14r)

29. This tracing shows a normal sinus rhythm. At first glance, there are inferior Q waves suggestive of an inferior infarct. However, the short PR interval and obvious delta waves in the anteroseptal leads are diagnostic of Wolff-Parkinson-White syndrome. There is an inferior pseudo-infarct pattern. Fusion complexes could be coded, since each QRS complex is a fusion between ventricular activation via the normal conduction pathway and via the bypass tract.

(Answers: 2a, 5a, 6h, 12g)

30-1; 30-2. These ECGs demonstrate pacemaker malfunction. The limb leads demonstrate sinus rhythm with criteria for left atrial abnormality. There is also first degree AV block and left bundle branch block. Rhythm strips

demonstrate ventricular pacing at 72 bpm. The third complex in rhythm strip 30-2 is a paced complex. However, the escape interval before the next QRS complex is greater than the paced interval, suggesting failure of the pacemaker to fire appropriately, probably the result of oversensing. At other times, the pacemaker fires prematurely, suggesting undersensing. Failure to sense appropriately is typical for lead insulation fracture. The last complex in the rhythm strips is probably a fusion beat between a paced and native QRS complex.

(Answers: 2a, 5a, 6a, 7f, 8b, 12g, 13b, 13g, 13h)

31. This tracing shows a sinus tachycardia with right axis deviation, right atrial abnormality, and absent R waves throughout the precordial leads. The findings are consistent with right ventricular hypertrophy and probable congenital heart disease (dextrocardia). Nonspecific repolarization abnormalities are noted. Low voltage is present in the limb leads only.

(Answers: 2d, 8a, 9a, 9d, 10c, 12c, 14k)

32. This ECG demonstrates a sinus rhythm with a nonspecific atrial abnormality and first degree AV block. Ventricular premature complexes are present, including one pair of VPCs. After the pair, a compensatory pause triggers a demand ventricular pacemaker that fires for two beats at approximately 60 bpm. The second of the paced beats is a fusion complex (the combination of a normal sinus beat and a ventricular paced beat). A right bundle branch block is present with secondary repolarization abnormalities and evidence for previous anteroseptal myocardial infarction. The first complex in leads V_4 through V_6 demonstrates a subtle aberration in the normal T wave configuration that is probably the result of the preceding ventricular premature complex. Remember to code for coronary artery disease and ventricular demand pacing.

(Answers: 2a, 4d, 5a, 6a, 7b, 8c, 11i, 12g, 12h, 13b, 14r)

33. This tracing demonstrates a sinus rhythm with an extensive acute anteroseptal, anterolateral, and high lateral myocardial infarction. Low voltage is present in both the limb and precordial leads. Remember to score ST segment changes consistent with myocardial injury and coronary artery disease.

(Answers: 2a, 11a, 11c, 11d, 12e, 14r)

34. This ECG shows an acute or recent inferior myocardial infarction with Q waves and ST segment elevation in leads III and aVF; associated marked ST segment depression is seen in the high lateral and precordial leads. The extensive ST segment depression and deep T wave inversion in the noninfarct leads suggest that a significant amount of ischemia is present in the myocardium remote from the infarct zone. Right atrial abnormality is present as well as ST segment abnormalities, suggesting myocardial injury and coronary artery disease. A nonspecific intraventricular conduction defect is present as well.

    (Answers: 2a, 7h, 8a, 11e, 12d, 12e)

35. This tracing shows a rapid wide complex rhythm with right axis deviation that is consistent with ventricular tachycardia. Electrical alternans is present, most apparent in lead V₂. Electrical alternans can be seen with tachycardias of either supraventricular or ventricular origin.

    (Answers: 4f, 9d, 9e)

36. This tracing demonstrates coarse atrial fibrillation with evidence for an old anteroseptal myocardial infarction with persisting ST segment elevation in leads V₂ through V₄. These findings are consistent with a chronic ventricular aneurysm. Nonspecific repolarization abnormalities are noted as well as evidence for coronary artery disease.

    (Answers: 2s, 11i, 11m, 12c, 14r)

37. This tracing shows a sinus rhythm with a pause secondary to a nonconducted atrial premature complex (manifest as a distortion of the baseline immediately following the T wave during the pause). Evidence for an old inferior infarction is noted with nonspecific repolarization abnormalities that are probably consistent with digitalis effect.

    (Answers: 2a, 2j, 11k, 12c, 14a)

38. This ECG demonstrates a markedly abnormal P wave axis with a PR interval of approximately 0.14 seconds. These findings are consistent with an ectopic atrial rhythm. The focus is probably low in the atrium, near the AV node, and effectively results in retrograde atrial activation. Because the PR interval

is greater than 0.11 seconds, it is classified as an ectopic atrial rather than a junctional rhythm.

    (Answers: 2g, 2t)

39. An underlying sinus rhythm is present on this tracing as well as a malfunctioning pacemaker with failure to sense. ST segment elevation is noted in leads I, aVL, V₂, and V₃, suggesting acute myocardial injury. Q waves are not present and thus definitive diagnosis for acute myocardial infarction cannot be made. The evidence is sufficient to warrant coding for coronary artery disease.

    (Answers: 2a, 12e, 13a, 13g, 14r)

40. The initial rhythm on this ECG is a sinus mechanism with first degree AV block. This is overridden by an accelerated idioventricular rhythm resulting in isorhythmic AV dissociation and fusion complexes. An atypical right bundle branch block is present that is most appropriately scored as a nonspecific intraventricular conduction defect with secondary repolarization abnormalities.

    (Answers: 2a, 4g, 5a, 5d, 6a, 7h, 12g)

41. This ECG demonstrates atrial fibrillation with left axis deviation, left anterior fascicular block, right bundle branch, and nonspecific repolarization abnormalities secondary to the intraventricular conduction defect. A single wide complex premature beat is noted. This most likely represents a ventricular premature contraction, as the initial QRS deflection is not identical to the native complex.

    (Answers: 2s, 7b, 7c, 9c, 12c)

42. This tracing demonstrates a wide complex tachycardia at 110 bpm. P waves are clearly visible in lead V₁ with evidence for left atrial abnormality and first degree AV block. Left axis deviation, left anterior fascicular block, and right bundle branch block are all present. Secondary repolarization abnormalities are also noted. Finally, Q waves are noted in leads V₁–V₄ and are diagnostic of old or age-indeterminate anteroseptal infarction.

    (Answers: 2d, 6a, 7b, 7c, 8b, 9c, 11i, 12g, 14r)

43. This ECG shows a sinus rhythm with normal variant early repolarization abnormalities (most prominent in leads II, III, aVF, V_5–V_6). Prominent peaked T waves are noted and are also consistent with a normal variant pattern.

(Answers: 1b, 2a, 12a, 12j)

44. This complex tracing from a patient with congenital heart disease shows atrial fibrillation with right axis deviation. Both right ventricular hypertrophy and left ventricular hypertrophy are apparent (combined ventricular hypertrophy) with secondary repolarization abnormalities. Although the tracing suggests possible old high lateral myocardial infarction with Q waves in leads I and aVL, this is a "pseudo-infarct" pattern on the basis of the congenital heart disease. A nonspecific intraventricular conduction defect is present.

(Answers: 2s, 7h, 9d, 10d, 12g)

45. This ECG shows a normal sinus rhythm with artifact due to tremor apparent in the limb leads. Although the QRS complexes are small, they do not meet formal criteria for low voltage as the total deflection of the QRS measures more than 5 mm. Left ventricular hypertrophy and secondary repolarization abnormalities are noted. A nonspecific intraventricular conduction defect is present (QRS duration >110 ms). The ST segment elevation in leads V_2 and V_3 is probably secondary to left ventricular hypertrophy. Very prominent U waves are present and the QT interval is prolonged. This patient developed torsades de pointes shortly after this tracing was acquired. The patient was markedly hypokalemic and hypomagnesemic and was on quinidine.

(Answers: 1d, 2a, 7h, 10b, 12g, 12k, 12l, 14c, 14f)

46. This tracing demonstrates a common technical error in the acquisition of the electrocardiogram. The ECG shows a normal sinus rhythm with inverted complexes in leads I and aVL with an otherwise normal tracing. This is due to incorrect electrode placement. Incidental findings include minor nonspecific repolarization abnormalities and probable left atrial enlargement.

(Answers: 1c, 2a, 8b, 12c)

47. Sinus bradycardia is noted with a nonspecific atrial abnormality. One aberrantly conducted atrial premature contraction is present. A normally functioning DDD pacemaker is noted with small ventricular spikes apparent in many of the leads (consistent with bipolar pacing). The pacemaker activity is most notable after the atrial premature complex in aVF. The escape complex was paced in both the atrium and the ventricle. The upstroke of the QRS complexes is markedly slurred in a pattern typical for Wolff-Parkinson-White syndrome, although this is nondiagnostic in the presence of ventricular pacing. Most of the complexes are pacemaker "pseudofusion" beats whereby a ventricular pacer spike occurs at the onset of the QRS but does not alter the usual conduction sequence (the patient's native unpaced QRS complexes were identical to those noted on this tracing). Left axis deviation is present as well as striking repolarization abnormalities that are probably most appropriately coded as secondary to intraventricular conduction defect or hypertrophy.

(Answers: 2c, 2k, 5a, 8c, 9c, 12g, 13e)

48. Close examination of this tracing reveals several important findings. A sinus tachycardia is present with first degree AV block and nonconducted atrial ventricular premature contractions. Rate-dependent intermittent left bundle branch block is present (manifest as normal ventricular conduction in complexes occurring after a pause). In spite of the intraventricular conduction delay with secondary repolarization abnormalities, an acute inferior myocardial infarction is apparent as evidenced by ST segment elevation and Q waves in leads II, III, and aVF.

(Answers: 2d, 2j, 6a, 7e, 7g, 11e, 12e, 14r)

49. This ECG shows a sinus rhythm with left ventricular hypertrophy, left atrial enlargement, and deeply inverted T waves with associated ST segment depression suggesting myocardial ischemia. In some leads (I and aVL), repolarization abnormalities are present that could be consistent with left ventricular hypertrophy-related changes. However, the ST-T findings in the right precordial leads strongly suggest associated ischemic heart disease. Prominent but nondiagnostic R waves are present in leads V_1–V_2.

(Answers: 2a, 8b, 10b, 12d)

50. This tracing demonstrates a normal sinus rhythm (with a rate just under 100 bpm). Q waves are present in leads II, III, aVF, and V_4–V_6 with prominent

R waves in leads V_1 and V_2. This pattern is diagnostic for old (or age-indeterminate) inferior, anterolateral, and posterior myocardial infarction. Left atrial enlargement and nonspecific repolarization abnormalities are also seen. These findings are consistent with coronary artery disease.

(Answers: 2a, 8b, 11g, 11k, 11l, 12c, 14r)

51. This is a markedly abnormal tracing showing a sinus tachycardia with prolonged first degree AV block (the P wave is partially hidden in the distal portion of the preceding T wave). ST segment elevation is present from V_1–V_5, suggesting an acute anteroseptal and anterior myocardial infarction. The QRS configuration changes for two beats (most apparent in aVL and aVF). This most likely represents a pair of premature ventricular complexes. Low voltage is present throughout both the limb and precordial leads. Remember also to code ST-T abnormalities suggesting myocardial injury and coronary artery disease.

(Answers: 2d, 4d, 6a, 9b, 11b, 11c, 12e, 14r)

52. This is an example of complete heart block with an underlying sinus rhythm showing ventriculophasic sinus arrhythmia. Note that the PP intervals containing a QRS are shorter than the PP intervals without a QRS. The escape rhythm is junctional. The P waves show evidence for right and left atrial abnormality. Criteria for left ventricular hypertrophy with secondary ST-T abnormalities are also met.

(Answers: 2a, 3d, 5e, 6e, 8a, 8b, 10b, 12g)

53. This ECG shows a sinus rhythm with right axis deviation and right atrial abnormality. An incomplete right bundle branch block is noted with a prominent R wave in the right precordial leads. All of these findings suggest right ventricular hypertrophy. A single ventricular premature contraction is present.

(Answers: 2a, 4a, 7a, 8a, 9d, 10c, 12g)

54. This tracing reveals sinus rhythm with atrial premature complexes and short nonsustained runs of atrial tachycardia with AV block. The second complex in the right precordial leads represents a fusion beat between an escape ventricular complex and a sinus beat. The fusion beat immediately follows a burst of atrial tachycardia with AV block. A delayed sinus node recovery time and nonspecific ST-T changes are present. These rhythm disorders are characteristic of sick sinus syndrome. Criteria for left ventricular hypertrophy are also noted.

(Answers: 2a, 2i, 2o, 4h, 5a, 6f, 10b, 12c, 14v)

55. This tracing demonstrates left ventricular hypertrophy with prominent voltage. Nonvoltage criteria for left ventricular hypertrophy also present on this ECG include: left axis deviation, left anterior fascicular block, nonspecific intraventricular conduction delay, delayed intrinsicoid deflection, nonspecific atrial abnormality, and secondary repolarization abnormalities including subtle ST segment elevation in leads V_2 and V_3.

(Answers: 2c, 7c, 7h, 8c, 9c, 10b, 12g)

56. This ECG shows sinus rhythm with left atrial enlargement, left axis deviation, left anterior fascicular block, and deeply inverted T waves that are suggestive of myocardial ischemia. Atrial premature complexes are noted. The first one is normally conducted and the second one is aberrantly conducted. The use of **14r**, coronary artery disease, for this tracing may seem reasonable in light of the ischemic-appearing T waves. However, coronary artery disease should be coded only when definite evidence (e.g., diagnostic Q waves, ischemic ST segment elevation) is present.

(Answers: 2a, 2i, 2k, 7c, 8b, 9c, 12d)

57. This tracing demonstrates a sinus rhythm. A prolonged QT interval is present with a prominent U wave in leads V_2 and V_3. Nonspecific repolarization abnormalities are also noted in the anterolateral leads. These findings are consistent with antiarrhythmic drug effect.

(Answers: 2a, 12c, 12k, 12l, 14c)

58. This is an example of atrial flutter with variable conduction. Nonspecific repolarization abnormalities are present. The R wave progression in the right precordial leads is delayed, although a tiny R wave is present in leads V_2 and V_3 and thus this does not qualify as an old anteroseptal infarct.

(Answers: 2r, 6f, 12c)

59. This tracing demonstrates an extensive myocardial infarction that is correctly coded as an acute anterior infarction (ST segment elevation and small Q waves in V_2 through V_5), and high lateral infarction (ST segment elevation and Q waves in I and aVL). There is normal sinus rhythm present as well as ST-T abnormalities suggestive of myocardial injury. Coronary artery disease should also be coded. Reciprocal changes are present, although this diagnosis is not an option on the score sheet.

(Answers: 2a, 11b, 11d, 12e, 14r)

60. This tracing shows a sinus rhythm with uniform fixed coupled ventricular premature contractions that are at times followed by a junctional escape rhythm. This results in AV dissociation for a short period of time. The junctional rhythm is termed "escape" rather than "accelerated" because the rate is ≤60 bpm. Evidence for a recent or acute inferior myocardial infarction is noted. Remember to code both ST-T changes suggesting injury and coronary artery disease.

(Answers: 2a, 3b, 4a, 5d, 11e, 12e, 14r)

61. This ECG shows atrial fibrillation with complete heart block and an accelerated junctional rhythm. A nonspecific intraventricular conduction defect is present as well as nonspecific repolarization abnormalities and prominent U waves. These findings are suggestive of digitalis toxicity. Hypokalemia can predispose to digitalis toxicity and also can cause prominent U waves.

(Answers: 2s, 3c, 6e, 7h, 12c, 12l, 14b, 14f)

62. This tracing shows an acute anterior and anterolateral myocardial infarction. Widespread ST segment elevation and PR depression are also present in leads I, II, III, and aVF. At the time that this tracing was taken, the patient was 36 hours post-infarction with a clinical scenario suggesting acute pericarditis (probably the result of transmural myocardial necrosis resulting in leakage of blood into the pericardial space causing acute inflammation). Left atrial enlargement is also noted as well as ventricular premature contractions, one of which is a fusion complex (the second beat in the right precordial leads).

(Answers: 2a, 4c, 5a, 8b, 11a, 11b, 12e, 12f, 14p, 14r)

63. Although at first glance this appears to be complete left bundle branch block, upon closer inspection we see that in the rhythm strip at the bottom of the tracing, a ventricular premature contraction resulted in a compensatory pause followed by a normally conducted sinus beat without evidence for left bundle branch block. Thus, this is sinus tachycardia with intermittent (rate-dependent) left bundle branch block. Secondary ST-T abnormalities and left atrial enlargement are also noted.

(Answers: 2d, 4a, 7g, 8b, 12g)

64. Atrial tachycardia with AV block is present. Mobitz type I (Wenckebach) second degree AV block is also noted intermittently on the tracing. The QRS complexes are variable and phasic; this pattern is consistent with electrical alternans. Nonspecific ST-T abnormalities are also present. High-voltage QRS complexes suggest left ventricular hypertrophy.

(Answers: 2o, 6b, 9e, 10a, 12c)

65. This ECG demonstrates a sinus rhythm with complete heart block. Ventricular pacing is noted throughout the tracing. The fine high frequency baseline artifact noted in the limb leads is probably secondary to a muscular tremor.

(Answers: 1d, 2a, 6e, 13d)

66. A sinus bradycardia is noted with left atrial enlargement and left ventricular hypertrophy. Extensive ST and T wave changes are noted, including deeply inverted T waves in I, aVL, and V_2–V_6. The magnitude of the T wave inversion suggests possible associated myocardial ischemia, although this is nondiagnostic in the presence of left ventricular hypertrophy.

(Answers: 2c, 8b, 10b, 12g)

67. This tracing was obtained at peak exercise and shows a sinus tachycardia at 151 bpm. Upsloping ST segment depression is present that is probably within normal limits and consistent with isolated J point depression. The tracing is otherwise within normal limits. This 50-year-old female was subsequently noted to have normal coronary arteries.

(Answers: 2d, 12i)

68. This ECG shows sinus tachycardia, right axis deviation, right bundle branch block, and secondary repolarization abnormalities. Although somewhat masked by the intraventricular conduction defect, ST segment elevation and Q waves suggesting acute anterior myocardial infarction are noted. Because the Q waves and ST segment elevation are present in leads V_1–V_5 as well as in leads I and aVL, correct diagnoses include acute anteroseptal, anterior, and high lateral myocardial infarction. A single atrial premature complex is noted; also remember to code for ST-T abnormalities suggesting myocardial injury and coronary artery disease.

(Answers: 2d, 2i, 7b, 9d, 11b, 11c, 11d, 12e, 14r)

69. This is an example of sinus bradycardia competing with a junctional escape mechanism resulting in AV dissociation and retrograde atrial activation. Normal variant early repolarization findings are also present.

(Answers: 2c, 2t, 3d, 5d, 12a)

70. The dominant finding on this tracing is that of an acute inferior myocardial infarction with Q waves and ST segment elevation in leads II, III, and aVF. The rhythm is sinus with a ventricular premature complex followed by a ventricular escape beat. Remember to code ST-T abnormalities suggesting myocardial injury and coronary artery disease.

(Answers: 2a, 4a, 4h, 11e, 12e, 14r)

71. This difficult tracing shows left bundle branch block with secondary ST-T abnormalities and atrial tachycardia (repetitive with short paroxysms). The escape complexes are probably junctional in origin with retrograde atrial activation. Highly unusual rhythm abnormalities such as this are seen commonly in patients with digitalis toxicity.

(Answers: 2m, 2t, 3b, 7f, 12g, 14b)

72. This tracing shows sinus tachycardia with markedly abnormal P waves suggesting both right and left atrial enlargement. The tracing also meets criteria for an old or age-indeterminate anteroseptal myocardial infarction (this can be a pseudo-infarct pattern in the setting of chronic obstructive pulmonary disease). A vertical axis is present that just barely meets criteria

for right axis deviation ($>+100°$). Nonspecific ST-T segment abnormalities are seen. Many of these features are characteristic of patients with chronic lung disease.

(Answers: 2d, 8a, 8b, 11i, 12c, 14m)

73. This ECG shows evidence for sinus bradycardia with marked left ventricular hypertrophy. Left axis deviation and left anterior fascicular block are present with repolarization abnormalities consistent with left ventricular hypertrophy (T wave inversion in the high lateral and lateral leads with ST segment elevation in leads V_1 through V_3). Prominent U waves are noted (commonly associated with left ventricular hypertrophy). A deep Q wave is present in lead aVL; this is a ''pseudo-infarct'' pattern. These findings are all consistent with the patient's history of hypertrophic cardiomyopathy.

(Answers: 2c, 7c, 9c, 10b, 12g, 12l, 14q)

74. This tracing shows a sinus tachycardia with left bundle branch block and secondary ST-T segment abnormalities. The ECG also meets criteria for both right and left atrial abnormality (the P wave is greater than 2.5 mm in amplitude in lead II with a prominent negative deflection of the terminal portion of the P wave in lead V_1).

(Answers: 2d, 7f, 8a, 8b, 12g)

75. This bizarre tracing is from a patient with profound hyperkalemia. The QRS is markedly prolonged (typically seen only when the potassium levels are severely elevated). The QT interval is prolonged. The underlying rhythm is atrial fibrillation and a ventricular pacemaker is present but is failing to capture and sense.

(Answers: 2s, 7h, 12k, 13f, 13g, 14e)

76. An acute inferior and posterior myocardial infarction is present on this ECG. This is manifest as ST segment elevation in leads II, III, and aVF (inferior infarct) with horizontal ST segment depression of approximately 2 mm in leads V_2 and V_3 with an early transition (posterior infarct). Other important findings include accelerated junctional tachycardia with an

underlying sinus rhythm and third degree AV block. These findings are consistent with coronary artery disease.

(**Answers: 2a, 3c, 6e, 11e, 11f, 12e, 14r**)

77. This tracing shows a sinus bradycardia with SA exit block (the pauses are approximately two times the normal R to R interval). Also noted are: ventricular premature complex, first degree AV block, nonspecific intraventricular conduction disturbance, and ST segment abnormalities secondary to the intraventricular conduction defect. SA exit block and first degree AV block are common findings in patients with sick sinus syndrome.

(**Answers: 2c, 2f, 4a, 6a, 7h, 12g, 14v**)

78. This ECG demonstrates a wide complex irregular rhythm at approximately 140 bpm. The intraventricular conduction defect is left bundle branch block but with secondary repolarization abnormalities. The Q waves in the anterior and inferior leads are of uncertain clinical significance in the presence of left bundle branch block. Low voltage is present in the limb leads only; left axis deviation is present.

(**Answers: 2s, 7f, 9a, 9c, 12g**)

79. This tracing shows a marked sinus bradycardia competing with a junctional escape rhythm at approximately 40 bpm. This competition results in AV dissociation. Evidence for an old anteroseptal myocardial infarction is noted with nonspecific repolarization abnormalities. Marked variation in the sinus rate is noted consistent with sinus arrhythmia.

(**Answers: 2b, 2c, 3b, 5d, 11i, 12c, 14r**)

80. This tracing shows a sinus tachycardia at 101 bpm. A nonspecific intraventricular conduction disturbance is present with evidence for left ventricular hypertrophy (the tallest R wave in lead aVL is 14 mm). Repolarization abnormalities consistent with a strain pattern are present. First degree AV block is also noted with a PR interval of approximately 205 ms. Q waves are noted in leads V_1–V_4 suggesting previous anteroseptal myocardial infarction. The QRS complexes are varying in amplitude (most prominent in lead III); this is an example of electrical alternans. Electrical alternans in this case is probably secondary to underlying hypertension and coronary artery disease.

(**Answers: 2d, 6a, 7h, 9e, 10b, 11i, 12g, 14r**)